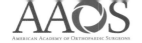

AAOS
AMERICAN ACADEMY OF ORTHOPAEDIC SURGEONS

ALS for the BLS Provider
Field Guide

Daniel E. Glick, BPS, AEMT-CC
Arthur Breault, NREMT-P, RN,

JONES AND BARTLETT PUB
Sudbury, Massachusetts
BOSTON   TORONTO   LONDON   SINGAPORE

Jones and Bartlett Publishers
World Headquarters
40 Tall Pine Drive
Sudbury, MA 01776
978-443-5000
info@jbpub.com
www.jbpub.com

Jones and Bartlett
Publishers Canada
6339 Ormindale Way
Mississauga, Ontario
L5V 1J2 Canada

Jones and Bartlett
Publishers International
Barb House, Barb Mews
London W6 7PA
United Kingdom

Production Credits
Publisher–Public Safety Group: Kimberly Brophy
Acquisition Editor–EMS: Christine Emerton
Associate Editor: Amanda Brandt
Senior Production Editor: Susan Schultz
Manufacturing Buyer: Therese Connell
Composition: NK Graphics
Cover and Text Design: Anne Spencer
Senior Photo Researcher and Photographer: Kimberly Potvin
Cover Image: © Photos.com
Printing and Binding: Imago
Cover Printing: Imago
ISBN-13: 978-0-7637-5171-5

6048

Printed in China
11 10 09 08 07   10 9 8 7 6 5 4 3 2 1

Contents

Acknowledgments

We would like to thank the following reviewers:

John R. Brophy
EMS Communications
 Supervisor and EMT-B
 Instructor
Liberty Health–Jersey
 City Medical Center
 EMS
Jersey City,
New Jersey

**Ginger K. Floyd, BA,
 NREMT-P**
Assistant Professor
Austin Community
 College
Austin, Texas

Martin Givens
Santa Monica USD/
 ROP
Los Angeles Valley
 College
Valley Glen, California

Steve Kelly, BS, EMT-P
Fire and EMS
 Instructor
West Chester Fire
 Department
West Chester, Ohio

**Brian Reiselbara, BA,
 NREMT-P, CCEMT-P**
Chief Flight
 Paramedic/Trainer
Maniilaq MedFlight
Kotzebue, Alaska

Craig Spector
President, 2007
 ECSI National Advisory
 Council
Chairman, CPR Heart
 Starters Inc.
 Safety Training
Warrington,
Pennsylvania

Jedediah O. Stancill, EMT-I
BLS Instructor
East Carolina Medical Transport, LLC
Snow Hill,
North Carolina

Tim Witten, CSP, CFPS, OHST, CHMM
EMT-B Instructor
Kentucky Fire and Safety Compliance
Bowling Green, Kentucky

Use of the Guide

This guide is designed to assist the user in recalling knowledge acquired or confirmed from other sources. We have attempted to be as accurate as possible and have taken care to make certain that all EMS references and drug information in this text are correct and compatible with national standards generally accepted at the time of publication. The American Academy of Orthopaedic Surgeons, the author, and publisher disclaim any liability, loss, injury, or damage incurred as a consequence, directly or indirectly, of the use and application of the contents of this book. The user is advised to carefully consult their medical director prior to making any deviations from locally accepted protocols and guidelines.

Writing in the Guide

For making permanent notes, use a felt-tip pen such as a Sharpie™ and allow the ink to dry thoroughly (may take as long as 30 minutes). For temporary notes, erase as soon as possible (within 10 minutes preferably) with alcohol.

■ Introduction

The *ALS for the BLS Provider Field Guide* is a tool that can be used by BLS providers to provide quality assistance to their ALS counterparts. Oftentimes, a BLS provider is left watching the "action" on scene while an ALS provider works; the information in this guide will facilitate BLS-ALS interaction on scene and ensure optimal patient care. This guide is intended to help first responders and EMT-Bs recognize, anticipate, and assist with the needs of ALS providers.

This guide requires appropriate training in prehospital emergency medicine and is not intended to be an exhaustive review. EMS providers are cautioned to adhere to their local EMS protocols and to seek advice from medical control as indicated. You are encouraged to confirm information in this guide with other sources, drug inserts, standards of care, and manufacturer literature for greater detail. The authors, AAOS, and publisher assume no liability with respect to the accuracy, completeness, or application of information in this field guide.

Advanced life support (ALS) is an essential level of prehospital medical care. Various indicators should prompt you to recognize patients in need of ALS care. It is important that every prehospital patient needing ALS care receive it without delay and that all patients are transported to definitive care at a hospital in a timely fashion. This may be accomplished either by intercepting with an ALS unit or by transport to an appropriate hospital, whichever can be effected more quickly.

■ ALS Assistance Guidelines

When to Call for ALS

- BLS unit shall not wait on scene for arrival of the ALS unit.
- Request for ALS should be made as soon as the patient's condition is recognized as needing ALS. This can sometimes be determined from dispatch information.
- The following conditions may warrant dispatch of an available ALS unit (consider simultaneous 9-1-1 dispatch):
  - Cardiac arrest
  - Chest pain
  - Stroke, onset within the last 2 hours
  - Respiratory arrest
  - Respiratory distress
  - Overdose
  - Unresponsive or altered mental status (AMS)

- Allergic reaction
- Diabetic reaction
- Serious trauma, penetrating trauma, burns > 15% BSA, chest, head
- Unstable vital signs
  - Blood pressure
    - Adult SBP < 90 mm Hg
    - Pediatric SBP < 70 to 80 mm Hg
    - Infant SBP < 60 mm Hg
  - Respiratory rate
    - Adult: Less than 10 breaths/min or greater than 30 breaths/min
    - Pediatric: Less than 10 breaths/min or greater than 60 breaths/min
    - Ineffective breathing, grunting, or stridor
- Emergency medical dispatch priority (Charlie/Delta/Echo)
- Anytime medications are going to be administered

When to Cancel ALS

- After completing the patient assessment and determining that a patient does not require the activation of an ALS intercept or ALS treatment in accordance with statewide treatment protocols

- When there is no foreseeable need for ALS treatment based on the patient's condition or mechanism of injury
- When it is determined that the patient can be transported to an appropriate health care facility in less time than it would take ALS to arrive on scene or intercept BLS during transport

Prehospital Care Reporting

- Ensure that all documentation is clear and easy to read.
- If documenting patient care for an ALS provider, have the ALS provider review documentation prior to submitting it to the hospital.
- *Do not sign* for any care that was not provided by you.
- Follow the prehospital care documentation algorithm.
- Follow all local and regional protocols for documenting care.

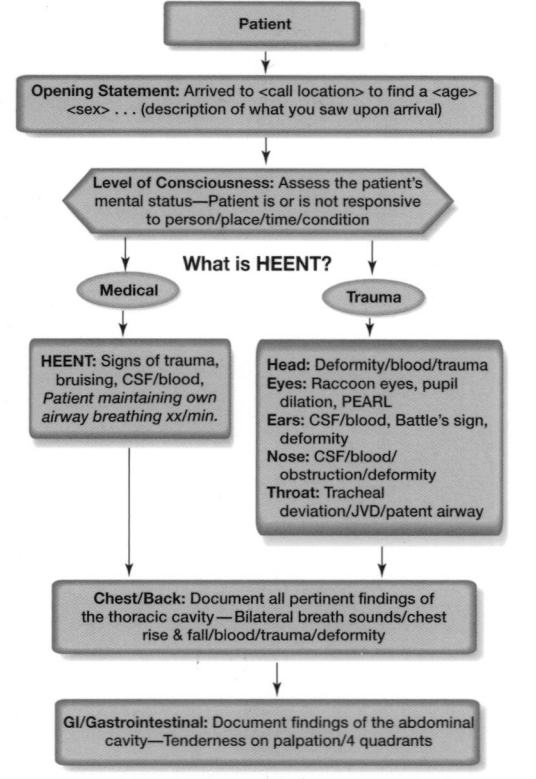

Patient

Opening Statement: Arrived to <call location> to find a <age> <sex> . . . (description of what you saw upon arrival)

Level of Consciousness: Assess the patient's mental status—Patient is or is not responsive to person/place/time/condition

What is HEENT?

Medical

Trauma

HEENT: Signs of trauma, bruising, CSF/blood, *Patient maintaining own airway breathing xx/min.*

Head: Deformity/blood/trauma
Eyes: Raccoon eyes, pupil dilation, PEARL
Ears: CSF/blood, Battle's sign, deformity
Nose: CSF/blood/obstruction/deformity
Throat: Tracheal deviation/JVD/patent airway

Chest/Back: Document all pertinent findings of the thoracic cavity—Bilateral breath sounds/chest rise & fall/blood/trauma/deformity

GI/Gastrointestinal: Document findings of the abdominal cavity—Tenderness on palpation/4 quadrants

GU/Gastro Urinary: Document any findings of the reproductive and waste disposal system. Do not examine or expose genitalia unless necessary. If no exam is performed, mark "No Exam."

↓

Extremities: Document any findings in all four extremities, designate specific extremity of finding (eg, ℝ Right arm or leg, Ⓛ left arm or leg, deformity, pulse, and neurologic exam)

↓

Skin: Note condition of skin, temperature, color, turgor, intact, lesions, etc.

↓

Treatment: List all treatment modalities used to include SpO$_2$, blood glucose, O$_2$ administration, ECG, etc.

↓

Closing Statement: Document all medication administration on continuation form. "A stable patient with . . . was turned over to <hospital>, report given." Initial at close of statement.

■ Radio Operations

If the ALS provider asks you to make a report to the hospital or medical director, gather and relay the following information about the patient:

- Age
- Gender
- Pertinent medical history
- Current chief complaint
- Current medications
- Last set of vital signs (blood pressure, pulse, respirations)
- Medications administered by medic
- Medications administered by order of online medical control
- Estimated time of arrival (ETA)

Keep the report brief and to the point.

At some point during the report, tell the medical director how long it will be until you will arrive at the facility. This may or may not change the medical director's decision or course of action.

You may be asked to provide additional medications that are not in protocol or on standing orders. If the medical director is on the line and you are not sure how to proceed, this is the time to request guidance.

Sample Radio Report

_____ this is ALS unit _____ inbound your facility with a _____ -year-old
(Hospital name/MD#)   (identifier/number)   (age)

_____ complaining of: _____
(male/female)   (Description of the reason why EMS was called and current
                                  subjective assessment)

Patient is currently taking: _____ with a history of: _____
                            (List pt medications)   (Detail pertinent medical history)

Last set of vital signs were: Pulse: _____ Respiration: _____ Blood pressure: _____ over _____
                                    (rate)   (resp/min)   (systolic/diastolic)

_____ showing on the monitor. Care by EMS included: _____
(ECG rhythm)   (Report all care administered by EMS, including medications)

Patient's current status is: _____
                            (Report patient's current status, (+) and (–) changes as a result of EMS care)

■ Abdominal Pain

Description Abdominal pain can arise from the tissues of the abdominal wall that surround the abdominal cavity and/or the organs within the abdominal cavity. These organs include the stomach, small intestine, colon, liver, gallbladder, and pancreas. Occasionally, pain may be felt in the abdomen even though it is arising from organs that are close to, but not within, the abdominal cavity; for example, the lower lungs, the kidneys, and the uterus or ovaries.

Abdominal pain can be:

- Sharp, dull, stabbing, cramplike, knifelike, or twisting
- Brief, lasting for a few minutes and then going away, or constant
- A symptom associated with transient disorders or serious disease

Due to the complexity of the abdomen, the focused history and physical exam are intended to identify a *degree of life-threat*, not a diagnosis.

Females of childbearing age *must* be assumed to be pregnant until a hospital test determines they are not, regardless of whether they are taking birth control pills or have had a tubal ligation. Think ectopic pregnancy.

Signs and Symptoms

- **Inflammation of the parietal peritoneum.** Pain is steady and aching and worsened by changes in the tension of the peritoneum caused by pressure or positional change. It is often accompanied by tension of the abdominal muscles contracting to relieve such tension.

- **Obstruction of the gastrointestinal tract.** Pain is often intermittent or "colicky."

- **Abdominal vascular disturbances (thrombosis or embolism).** Pain can be sudden or gradual in onset and can be severe or mild.

- **Rupture of an abdominal aortic aneurysm.** Pain may radiate to the back, flank, or genitals.

- **Referred pain.** Pain that is felt in the abdomen may be "referred" from elsewhere (eg, a disease process in the chest may cause pain in the abdomen). Abdominal processes can cause radiated pain elsewhere (eg, gallbladder pain—in cholecystitis or cholelithiasis—is often referred to the shoulder).

- Use OPQRST, SAMPLE.

Medical

ALS for the BLS Provider

- Apply oxygen via nonrebreathing mask.
- Consider possibility of fluid loss.
- Prepare IV supplies. Two sets of tubing and preparation kits might be needed.

Key Questions

- Is there any associated pain?

  If so:

  - Time of onset?
  - Where is the pain located?
  - Does the pain radiate?
  - On a scale from 1 to 10, how severe is the pain?
  - Has the patient had a fever associated with the condition?

- Is there a possibility of pregnancy? Date of last menses?

  - Consider ectopic pregnancy.

- Has there been any penile/vaginal or rectal bleeding/discharge?

- When was the last time the patient ate?

- Are there any signs/symptoms of trauma?

Other Considerations

- Inflammation
- Infection (appendicitis, pelvic inflammatory disease)

- Gastric/peptic ulcer
- Perforation
- Bowel obstruction
- Diverticulitis
- Gastroenteritis
- Pregnancy (ectopic)
- Pneumonia
- Gynecologic etiology
- Atypical myocardial infarction (heart attack)

Gastrointestinal Bleeding

Description Form of hemorrhage (loss of blood) in the gastrointestinal tract, from the pharynx to the rectum. The degree of bleeding can range from nearly undetectable to acute, massive, and life threatening.

Signs and Symptoms

- Coffee-ground emesis; frank bleeding; dark, tarry stools; bleeding complications due to the use of heparin, aspirin, clopidogrel (Plavix). Secondary to complications of renal failure.
- Can be minor or life threatening.
- Can be obvious or subtle.
- Produces a wide variety of presentations.

ALS for the BLS Provider

- Apply oxygen via nonrebreathing mask.
- Apply cardiac monitor.
- Monitor blood pressure.
- Set up IV supplies.

The ALS provider will support ventilation and oxygenation, and provide fluid support. Systolic blood pressure > 90 mm Hg must be maintained, and ECG monitored.

Key Questions

- What is the patient's medication history?
- What does the blood look like (color and amount)?
- What do the stools/bowel movement look like (color)? Is blood present?
- What are the patient's vital signs when standing and lying down?

Other Considerations

- Overuse of nonsteroidal anti-inflammatory drugs
- Lesion or malignancy
- Stomach infection

Abdominal Aortic Aneurysm

Description The term *abdominal aortic aneurysm* (AAA) is used to describe a localized dilation of the abdominal aorta. Risk factors include hypertension and male gender. AAAs are commonly divided according to their size and symptoms. An aneurysm is usually considered to be present if the measured outer aortic diameter is greater than 3 cm. The progression is of increasing diameter over time, followed eventually by the development of symptoms (usually rupture). If the outer diameter exceeds 5 cm, the aneurysm is considered to be large.

Signs and Symptoms The clinical manifestation of a ruptured AAA can include a pulsatile mass, and low back, flank, abdominal, or groin pain. Bleeding usually leads to hypoperfusion, shock with hypotension, tachycardia, cyanosis, and altered mental status.

Medical

ALS for the BLS Provider

- Provide high-concentration oxygen via nonrebreathing mask.
- Prepare IV administration supplies (two sets).
- Prepare for possible pressure infusion (wrap blood pressure cuff around IV bag).
- Monitor with 12-lead ECG.
- Elevate foot end of stretcher—position for shock.
- Check pulse oximetry.

Key Questions

- Can the patient describe the pain?
- Is it getting worse?
- Are there distal pulses? Are the extremities mottled or discolored?
- Has the patient ever had an aneurysm? What size?
- Has the patient had abdominal surgeries in the past? Look at the abdomen for old scars.

Other Considerations

- Retroperitoneal bleeding
- Infection/sepsis
- Trauma
- Adhesions from previous abdominal surgeries

■ Altered Mental Status

Description An altered mental status can come about accidentally or intentionally through indigestion, fever, sleep deprivation, psychiatric condition, starvation, oxygen deprivation, nitrogen narcosis (deep diving), a traumatic accident, and the ingestion of alcohol, opioids, or certain plants.

Signs and Symptoms Signs and symptoms of altered mental status may include dreams;

euphoria; ecstasy; psychosis, as well as purported premonitions; appearance of intoxication; sleepiness; changes in personality, and complete unresponsiveness.

ALS for the BLS Provider

- Apply oxygen. Patient may not be able to tolerate the nonrebreathing mask; consider nasal canula at 6 L/min.
- Check blood glucose (if local protocols allow).
- Prepare IV supplies.
- Apply 12-lead ECG as soon as possible and run strips.
- Gather supplies and equipment necessary for ALS provider to administer D_{50} IV or glucagon IM for administration.
- Repeat Glasgow Coma Scale, neurologic exam, and/or blood glucose.

Key Questions

- Can you rule out head injury, infection, cerebrovascular accident (CVA), overdose, or seizure?
- Was the onset of altered mental status sudden or gradual?
- Signs of neurologic posturing, incontinence, or neck rigidity?

Medical

- Can you rule out infectious disease, such as meningitis?
- When was the last time the patient ate? What was it?
- Are there any clues in the surrounding environment?

Other Considerations

- **Vascular thrombosis.** Hemorrhage, mass effect, pupils
- **Hydrocephalus.** Tumor, infection, meningitis, encephalitis, any recent illness, fever, or neck rigidity
- **Seizure.** Trauma, epilepsy, past medical history, medications, mechanism of injury
- **Diabetes.** Hypoglycemia, diabetic ketoacidosis, hyperosmolar hyperglycemic nonketotic coma (HHNC)
- **Environment.** Heat exhaustion, heat stroke, hypothermia, activity, intake
- **Recreational substances.** Opiates, alcohol, medications
- **HazMat.** Carbon monoxide
- **Sepsis.** Shock
- **Psychiatric.** Schizophrenia, depression, acute psychosis

■ Allergy/Anaphylaxis

Description An *allergy* is an abnormally high sensitivity to certain substances, such as pollens, foods, or microorganisms. Common indications of allergy include sneezing, itching, and skin rashes. *Anaphylaxis* is a sudden, severe allergic reaction characterized by a sharp drop in blood pressure, urticaria, and breathing difficulties that is caused by exposure to a foreign substance, such as a drug or bee venom, after a preliminary or sensitizing exposure. The reaction may be fatal if emergency treatment, including epinephrine injections, is not given immediately.

Signs and Symptoms

- **Skin.** Itching; hives (red, itchy, possibly raised patches); flushing skin; swelling of the face, neck, hands, feet, or tongue; warm, tingling feeling in the face, mouth, chest, feet, and hands

- **Respiratory.** Feeling of tightness in throat or chest, coughing, increased work of breathing, labored noisy breathing, hoarseness to a loss of voice, stridor (high-pitched sound during inspirations), wheezing

- **Cardiac.** Increased heart rate and low blood pressure

Medical

- **Other.** Itchy, watery eyes; headache; runny nose
- **Progression to shock.** Altered mental status; flushed and dry or pale, cool, and clammy skin; nausea and vomiting; changes in vital signs; and a feeling of impending doom verbalized by the patient

ALS for the BLS Provider

- Apply oxygen via nonrebreathing mask.
- Prepare IV supplies. Two sets of tubing and preparation kits might be needed.
- Apply pulse oximeter.
- Locate and gather diphenhydramine and epinephrine for administration by ALS provider.
- If SpO$_2$ drops below 95%, prepare endotracheal intubation tools for ALS provider.

Key Questions

- Was the onset gradual or sudden?
- What was the patient exposed to?
- Type of reaction? Previous reactions?
- Rash, itching, or swelling?
- Noticeable sting/bite marks?
- Swelling of the face or tongue? Difficulty breathing?
- Medical alert tag indicating allergies?

- Does the patient have his or her own medications (eg, an EpiPen)? Follow local protocol for BLS administration of EpiPen, if applicable.
- Noticeable lung sounds (wheezing, congested)?

Other Considerations

- Chemical exposure
- Latex allergy
- Sepsis/infection
- Acute respiratory distress syndrome

■ COPD and CHF Exacerbation

Description *Chronic obstructive pulmonary disease* (COPD) is a disorder marked by persistent obstruction of bronchial air flow. It is characterized by difficulty breathing, wheezing, and a chronic cough. *Congestive heart failure* (CHF) is a condition marked by weakness, edema, and shortness of breath. It is caused by the inability of the heart to maintain adequate blood circulation in the peripheral tissues and the lungs.

Signs and Symptoms

- Chronic lung disease associated with smoking history
- Cardiac history complicated by COPD, noncompliance with medications

Medical

- Cardiac history, diuretic medications, digitalis, ACE inhibitors
- Peripheral edema and jugular vein distension (JVD)
- Poor activity tolerance
- Emphysema (thin, barrel-chested, wheezing, productive cough, normal SpO_2)
- Bronchitis (obese, wheezing, productive cough, low SpO_2)
- Lung sounds congested and/or decreased
- Sputum: CHF clear to pink frothy; COPD white, yellow, green, may become thick/sticky

COPD AND CHF

COPD	CHF
• Increased shortness of breath, shortness of breath during exertion • Progressively gets worse • Coughing • Change in sputum color and thickness	• Shortness of breath (dyspnea) • Sudden onset • Coughing • Pulmonary congestion • Jugular vein distention • Inability to lie flat • Distended abdomen

ALS for the BLS Provider

- Provide high-concentration oxygen via nonrebreathing or bag-mask device.
- Set up suction equipment. Be prepared to suction.
- Apply pulse oximetry and end-tidal CO_2 monitoring equipment.
- Prepare for IV fluid administration.
- Allow patient to sit in a position of comfort.
- Ready the following medications for administration by ALS provider:
  - Albuterol/ipratropium (Atrovent) (nebulized)
  - Furosemide (Lasix)
  - Nitroglycerin

Other Considerations

- Pneumonia
- Asthma
- Allergies

Key Questions

- Was the onset sudden or gradual?
- If the answers to the following questions are positive, the patient likely has CHF.
  - History of congestive heart failure?
  - Rales on lung examination?
  - Edema to legs?

Medical

- Any previous history of intubation or mechanical ventilation?

■ Cardiac Emergencies

Chest Pain/Acute Coronary Syndrome (ACS)

Description Chest pain is a common symptom that can be caused by many different conditions. Some causes of chest pain, such as angina, heart attack, or tearing of the aorta, require prompt medical attention. The most serious complication is a chaotic arrhythmia called *ventricular fibrillation*, for which an AED should be readied and/or available. Other causes of chest pain can be evaluated electively, such as spasm of the esophagus, gallbladder attack, or inflammation of the chest wall. Therefore, an accurate diagnosis is important in providing proper treatment to patients with chest pain.

Signs and Symptoms

- Gradual versus sudden onset, activity at the time
- Worsens when lying down
- Changes with respiratory movement
- ECG changes
- Pain not relieved by antacids
- Pain worsens with exercise, not relieved by rest or nitroglycerin

- Elderly female might not present with typical findings
- History of hypertension, type 2 diabetes

The risk factors for atherosclerosis are generally similar to the risk factors for myocardial infarction:

- Older age
- Male gender
- Cigarette smoking
- High cholesterol
- Diabetes
- High blood pressure
- Obesity

Cardiac-type chest pain:

- Chest pain is the most common symptom of acute myocardial infarction and is often described as a sensation of tightness, pressure, or squeezing.
- Pain radiates most often to the left arm, but can also radiate to the lower jaw, neck, right arm, back, and epigastrium, where it may mimic heartburn.
- Shortness of breath (dyspnea)
- Diaphoresis (an excessive form of sweating)
- Lightheadedness, nausea, vomiting, and palpitations

ALS for the BLS Provider

- Apply oxygen. Patient may not be able to tolerate nonrebreathing mask; consider nasal cannula at 6 L/min.
- Apply 12-lead ECG as soon as possible and run strips as often as every 5 minutes.
- Prepare IV supplies.
- Prepare the following medications for administration by ALS provider (BLS administration if local protocols allow):
  - Nitroglycerin
  - Aspirin
- Print a reading of the ECG immediately for interpretation by the ALS provider.
- ST elevation needs to be reported to the ALS provider immediately.
- Prepare IV fluid and tubing.
- Prepare to supply the ALS provider with appropriate cardiac medications (ie, aspirin, nitroglycerin).
- Prepare to assist with advanced airway techniques.
- Consider transport to a facility capable of performing interventional cardiology.
- Early notification of ST elevation myocardial infarction (STEMI) patient.
- Prepare to perform CPR.

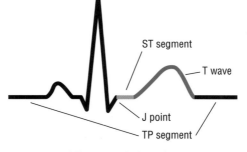

ST segment elevation

Key Questions

- Did the pain start with activity or rest?
- How does the patient describe the pain?
- Where is the pain?
- Does the pain radiate?
- Previous or similar episodes?
- Is there anything that makes the pain go away?
- What is the patient's medical history?
- Family history of cardiac issues?
- Are any of the following symptoms present?

Medical

- Sweating
- Nausea/vomiting
- Ankle swelling, fainting
- Have you contacted the hospital to make early notification of a patient with cardiac-related chest pain?

Other Considerations

- Myocardial infarction
- Congestive heart failure
- Pulmonary edema
- Pneumothorax
- Pericarditis
- GI disturbance
- Musculoskeletal discomfort
- Pneumonia
- Bronchitis
- Pulmonary embolism
- Aortic dissection

Cardiac Arrest

Description Cardiac arrest can be caused by any of the following:

- Hypoxia
- Hypothermia
- Overdose
- Pulmonary embolism

- Stroke
- Drowning
- Myocardial infarction
- Trauma

In your assessment, it is important to verify the following:

- Unresponsive
- Apnea
- No pulse

ALS for the BLS Provider

- Apply oxygen via nonrebreathing mask.
- Prepare two large-bore IVs.
  - 18 or 16 gauge
  - Macro-drip tubing with at least 1,000 mL normal saline bags
- Prepare endotracheal intubation equipment. Ask ALS provider preference for size, blade, and tube.
  - The following can be used on difficult airways:
    - Combitube
    - Laryngeal mask airway (LMA)
- Prepare suction device.
- Prepare to communicate information between paramedic and physician.
- Assist or apply cardiac monitor as soon as possible.

Medical

General Guidelines

- Request ALS early!
- Supply good, effective CPR. Limit interruptions of compressions, even when going down stairs.
- If witnessed arrest, apply AED immediately.
- If unwitnessed arrest, continue CPR for 2 minutes, then apply AED.
- Plan rhythm and pulse checks.
- Check pulses.
- Continuous CPR with an advanced airway in place.
- Good airway management. Don't hyperventilate.
- For dysrhythmia, apply AED.

Withholding Resuscitation

- Rigor mortis
- Dependent lividity
- Decapitation, decomposition, incineration
- Valid advanced directive

Always follow local protocols related to termination of resuscitation. Support the family or others after termination of resuscitation. Coordinate with law enforcement as required. Transport the remains to the closest appropriate facility.

Key Questions

- Pre-arrest events: What was the patient doing? When was the patient last seen?
- Was there any bystander CPR?
- How long has the patient been unconscious/unresponsive?
- Are there any advanced directives? DNR, living will, health care proxy?

■ Diabetic Emergencies

Description *Hypoglycemia* means low blood glucose. Blood glucose levels in healthy individuals fluctuate depending on the duration of fasting, meals, and activity. The normal range is 70 to 120 mg/dL. *Hyperglycemia* is a condition characterized by abnormally high levels of blood glucose, usually over 250 mg/dL.

Signs and Symptoms Hypoglycemia causes the body to release adrenaline. The released adrenaline causes symptoms of nervous system stimulation, such as anxiety, sweating, tremors, palpitations, nausea, and pallor. Hypoglycemia also starves the brain of glucose energy, which is essential for proper brain function. Lack of glucose energy to the brain can cause symptoms ranging from headache, mild confusion, and abnormal behavior to loss of consciousness, seizure, and coma. Severe hypoglycemia can

Medical

cause death. Symptoms of hypoglycemia occur at different levels of blood glucose in different patients. In most healthy individuals, symptoms of hypoglycemia might not occur until the glucose level drops below 65 mg/dL. Onset is sudden.

Hyperglycemia presents with frequent urination and increased thirst. Any of the following symptoms might be present: flushed face, dry skin, dry mouth, headache, abdominal pain, nausea and vomiting, drowsiness and lethargy, blurred vision, fruity-smelling breath, rapid heartbeat, and deep and labored breathing. Onset takes hours to days.

ALS for the BLS Provider

- Apply oxygen via nonrebreathing mask.
- Prepare IV supplies. Two sets of tubing and preparation kits might be needed.
  - Large-bore catheter; if possible, 18 gauge or higher
- Draw blood glucose reading if local protocol allows.
- If blood glucose is below 70 and the patient is oriented, give instant glucose by mouth.
- If blood glucose is below 70 and the patient presents with altered mental status, assist with preparation of dextrose 25 g, 50%, for ALS provider.
- If blood glucose is below 70 and you are unable to establish peripheral IV, prepare 1 mg glucagon IM for ALS provider.

Key Questions

- Was the onset of symptoms gradual or sudden?
- Increased thirst, hunger, or urination?
- Mental status changes (AVPU, GCS)?
- Medications? Insulin or pills? Compliance?
- Recent illness, infection, nausea, vomiting, or diarrhea?
- What is the patient's blood glucose level?
- When was the patient's last meal?
- Recheck blood glucose (if local protocol allows).

Other Considerations

- Stroke
- Overdose
- Trauma (closed head injury)
- Hypoxia
- Infection or sepsis
- Intoxication

■ OB/GYN Emergencies

Gynecologic Emergencies

Description Gynecologic emergencies include vaginal bleeding, pelvic inflammatory disease (PID), trauma, and sexual assault.

Signs and Symptoms

- Abnormal bleeding, menses
- Lower abdominal discomfort
- Vaginal discharge
- Vaginal bleeding—assume pregnant until hospital draws blood work
- Lower back pain
- Fever, chills, nausea, vomiting
- History of unprotected sex
- IUD use for birth control
- Cuts or tears of the vagina or rectum area
- Swelling or bruising for 2 to 3 days between the patient's legs

ALS for the BLS Provider

- Provide supplemental oxygen.
- Attempt to determine if pregnant, last day of menstrual period.
- Estimate pad count, apply pad to perineum to control bleeding.
- Place the patient in a position of comfort.
- Reassess vital signs, check for shock.
- Prepare for IV.
- Position for shock, feet elevated.
- Contact law enforcement if domestic violence or abuse is suspected.

• Do not let the patient wash or shower. Place any clothes worn during or right after an assault in a paper bag. The police may use them to get evidence.

Key Questions

- Date of last menses?
- Sudden or gradual onset?
- Any pain? Location of pain?
- Any bleeding or discharge? Heavy?
- Number of menstrual pads used prior to EMS arrival?
- Previous pregnancies?
- Does the patient exhibit any of the following signs?
  • Fever?
  • Chills?
  • Discharge? Color?
- Does the patient experience pain with intercourse?
- Any swelling of extremities, visual disturbances, headache?

Other Considerations

- UTI
- Miscarriage
- Appendicitis, right upper quadrant pain

Medical

- Endometriosis
- Gastroenteritis
- Rupture of ovarian cyst, sudden onset of mid-cycle pain
- Ovarian torsion
- Ectopic pregnancy
- Diverticular disease
- Hypothyroidism
- Blood clotting disorder
- Uterine fibroids
- Cervical or uterine cancer
- Hormone replacement therapy

Obstetric Emergencies

Description *Childbirth* is a natural process that usually takes place without complications. Assist the mother in the delivery of the baby. Determine whether transport should be immediate or if birth is imminent. Evaluate both mother and infant for complications, such as breech or limb presentation, prolapsed cord, premature birth, or meconium staining.

Predelivery emergencies also are possible, including ectopic pregnancy, excessive bleeding, abortion, and seizures.

Signs and Symptoms Childbirth usually begins spontaneously, following about 280 days after conception, but it may be started by artificial means if the pregnancy continues past 42 weeks gestation. The average length of labor is about 14 hours for a first pregnancy and about 8 hours in subsequent pregnancies. However, many women experience a much longer or shorter labor.

Labor can be described in terms of a series of phases:

- **Stage 1.** The cervix dilates (opens) from 0 to 10 cm. Contractions increase in strength as labor progresses.

- **Stage 2.** This stage starts when the baby enters the birth canal and ends when the baby is born. Uterine contractions become stronger. *Crowning* occurs when the top of the baby's head appears at the opening of the vagina.

- **Stage 3.** In this final stage, the placenta is pushed out of the vagina by the continuing uterine contractions. It is important that the entire placenta be removed from the uterus. If it is not, the uterine bleeding that is normal after delivery may be much heavier.

The following are potential obstetric complications:

- **Breech presentation.** This refers to the position of the baby in the uterus such that it will be delivered buttocks first, as opposed to the normal head-first position.

- **Prolapsed umbilical cord.** This occurs when the umbilical cord is pushed into the vagina ahead of the baby. The cord becomes compressed, cutting off blood flow to the baby.

- **Premature birth.** An infant who weighs less than 5.5 lb at birth or who is born before 36 weeks is considered premature.

- **Ectopic pregnancy.** The fertilized egg implants in a location outside the uterus and begins to develop there. The most common site is the fallopian tube, the tube that normally carries eggs from the ovary to the uterus. However, ectopic pregnancy can also occur in the ovary, the abdomen, and the cervical canal (the opening from the uterus to the vaginal canal). The fallopian tube is too narrow for the growing fetus. Eventually, the thin walls of the tube stretch and may burst (rupture), resulting in severe bleeding and possibly the death of the mother. Early symptoms include:

  - Fatigue
  - Nausea

- Missed period
- Breast tenderness
- Low back pain
- Mild cramping on one side of the pelvis
- Abnormal vaginal bleeding (usually spotting)
- If the tube has ruptured, blood may irritate the diaphragm and cause shoulder pain.

- **Placenta previa.** This occurs when the placenta is formed too low, close to the cervical opening, and will not allow for a normal delivery. This causes excessive prebirth bleeding and may be painless. Typically, this becomes a problem only in the third trimester.

- **Abruptio placenta.** This occurs when the placenta separates from the uterine wall, causing prebirth bleeding. Typically, this becomes a problem only in the third trimester.

- **Preeclampsia.** This is a complication of pregnancy and involves retention of fluid and hypertension. It may progress to seizures and/or coma.

ALS for the BLS Provider

- Apply oxygen via nonrebreathing mask to mother.
- Prepare OB kit for utilization.
- Prepare for rapid transport.
- Prepare for neonatal CPR.
- Prepare child/infant endotracheal intubation kit.

Key Questions

- General precautions and questions:
  - Date of last menses, estimated date of conception, weeks of gestation?
  - Sudden or gradual onset?
  - Any pain?
    - Location of pain?
  - Any bleeding or discharge?
    - Heavy?
  - Number of menstrual pads used prior to EMS arrival?
  - Previous pregnancies?
  - Does the patient exhibit any of the following signs?
    - Fever?
    - Chills?
    - Discharge? Color?
  - Does the patient experience pain with intercourse?

- Any swelling of extremities, visual disturbances, headache?
- Is the baby crowning?
- Treatment of birth complications:
  - **Delivery.** Control delivery; do not let the infant come out too quickly.
    - Suction mouth then nose, clamp, cut, and keep cord.
    - If the infant is warm and dry, give to the mother.
  - **Cord presentation.** Knee-chest position, hold pressure on baby's head, check pulse in cord, rapid transport.
  - **Cord around neck.** Unwrap cord from around neck and deliver.
  - **Breech.** Support presenting part, mother in Trendlenburg, knee-chest position, rapid transport.

Medical

APGAR SCALE

APGAR	Points	Score (1 min)	Score (5 min)
A—Appearance		___	___
Blue or pale extremities	0		
Pink trunk and blue extremities	1		
Completely pink	2		
P—Pulse		___	___
Absent	0		
< 100	1		
> 100	2		
G—Grimace		___	___
No response	0		
Grimace or whimpers	1		
Active/strong cry	2		
A—Activity (Muscle Tone)		___	___
Flaccid, limp	0		
Flexion	1		
Active motion	2		
R—Respiratory		___	___
Absent	0		
Slow, irregular	1		
Strong cry	2		
Total Score		___	___

■ Pediatric Emergencies

Description With regard to pediatric patients, the provider should pay particular attention to the following conditions: Hypoperfusion, protecting from hypothermia/heat loss, respiratory disorders/distress (croup, epiglottitis), fever/sepsis, meningitis, diarrhea and vomiting, altered mental status, poisoning, near-drowning, special needs considerations, and child abuse/neglect.

ALS for the BLS Provider

- Provide high-flow oxygen via nonrebreathing mask.
- Prepare equipment for ALS to perform blood glucose test on any pediatric patient exhibiting altered mental status.
- Special considerations:
  - Children compensate well for long periods of time and then crash without notable signs and symptoms.
  - On respiratory patients, beware of foreign objects lodged in trachea.
  - Protect the airway.
  - Respiratory arrest/distress causes *most* cardiac issues in pediatrics; determine cause of respiratory issues first.

Medical

Key Questions

- Is the patient's airway obstructed by a foreign body?
- Was the onset gradual or sudden? What was the history of events?
- Any drooling, fever/chills, recent illnesses?
- Work of breathing, nasal flaring?
  - Retractions, rate, tidal volume, ability to speak
  - Positioning (tripod)
- Bradycardia present? Bradycardia means hypoxia.
- Heart rate? Capillary refill?
- Assess mentation. What is the patient's baseline? Does the child recognize his or her parents?
  - Is mentation appropriate for developmental age?
- Recent intake? Diaper change frequency?
- Temperature? Last acetaminophen or ibuprofen? Dose?
- Any rash? Bruising? Immunization status?
- What is the child's blood glucose level? Level of oxygen saturation (if local protocol allows)?
- Is the story consistent with the injury? Was there a delay in seeking medical care? Is the injury pattern suggestive of abuse?

Other Considerations Consider hypoxia, toxic exposure, sepsis, abuse.

■ Pulmonary Emboli

Description Pulmonary embolism is an obstruction of a blood vessel in the lungs, usually due to a blood clot. Pulmonary embolism is a fairly common condition, and it can be fatal. It occurs when emboli block a pulmonary artery, usually due to a blood clot that breaks off from a large vein and travels to the lungs. Emboli can also be comprised of fat, air, or tumor tissue.

Signs and Symptoms

- Labored breathing, sometimes accompanied by chest pain
- Rapid pulse
- Cough that produces bloody sputum
- Low fever
- Fluid build-up in the lungs
- Less common symptoms include:
  - Coughing up a lot of blood
  - Pain caused by movement
  - Leg swelling
  - Bluish skin
  - Fainting
  - Swollen neck veins
- In some cases there are no symptoms.

Medical

ALS for the BLS Provider

- Provide supplemental oxygen.
- For low oxygen saturations: 95%; support ventilation and oxygenation.
- Support airway.
- Rule out other causes.
- Pertinent negatives: Pregnancy, prolonged immobilization, recent fractures
- Prepare equipment for fluid support.

Other Considerations Rule out acute myocardial infarction, other cardiac diseases, atrial fibrillation, COPD, pneumonia, and pneumothorax.

Key Questions

- Recent immobilization or surgeries?
- Hormone replacement medication or birth control medication?
- Past medical history of clots in the legs? History of varicose veins, venous stasis?
- Recent long bone fractures?
- Pregnancy?

■ Respiratory Distress

Description Respiratory distress involves difficulty in breathing that is often associated with lung or heart disease and that results in shortness of breath. It is also called *air hunger*. It is a common symptom of numerous medical disorders. The experience of dyspnea depends on the severity and underlying causes of the respiratory distress.

Symptoms The feeling itself results from a combination of impulses relayed to the brain from nerve endings in the lungs, rib cage, chest muscles, or diaphragm, combined with the patient's perception and interpretation of the sensation. In some cases, the patient's sensation of breathlessness is intensified by anxiety about its cause. Patients describe dyspnea variously as unpleasant shortness of breath, a feeling of increased effort or tiredness in moving the chest muscles, a panicky feeling of being smothered, or a sense of tightness or cramping in the chest wall.

Medical

ALS for the BLS Provider

- Apply pulse oximeter. If less than 95% SpO_2, and if patient is symptomatic, apply oxygen via nonrebreathing mask.
- Prepare to assist ventilation with bag-mask device if SpO_2 does not come up.
- Apply 12-lead ECG as soon as possible and run strips. Remember that an atypical myocardial infarction may present with no chest pain (eg, in elderly, female, diabetic).
- Prepare nebulizer.
- Assist with preparation of CPAP machine, if equipped.

Key Questions

- What was the patient doing during onset of symptoms?
- Was the onset gradual or sudden?
- Change in shortness of breath with lying flat?
- Is the patient able to speak?
- Significant work of breathing noted?
- Any previous episodes? Any pain?
- How many pillows are necessary to elevate the head so the patient can sleep?
- Is the difficulty any worse at night?
- Fever? Cough? Any change in sputum color?
- Is there any history of:
  - Lung disease?
  - Myocardial infarction, CHF, CAD, angina, bypass surgery?
  - Pneumonia?
  - HTN?
- Has the patient been intubated before?
- What medications is the patient taking (inhalers, diuretics, cardiac)?
- Is the patient becoming exhausted during evaluation?

Other Considerations

- COPD
- CHF

- Allergy
- Trauma
- Infection
- Anaphylactic shock
- Acute pneumonia
- Hemorrhage from the lungs
- Severe bronchospasms associated with asthma
- Cardiovascular diseases (myocardial infarction, pulmonary emboli, valvular problem)
- Neuromuscular disorders
- Hyperthyroidism or hypothyroidism
- Gastroesophageal reflux disease (GERD)
- Chronic anxiety disorders
- Obesity

Medical

■ Seizures

Description A seizure is a sudden attack, tonic-clonic body or repetitive movements (eg, eye blinking or lip smacking) or convulsion, as in epilepsy. May also present as a sudden onset or sensation of feeling or emotion.

Signs and Symptoms *Focal seizures* are classified as simple or complex based on the level of consciousness (wakefulness) during an attack. Simple partial seizures occur in patients who are conscious; complex partial seizures demonstrate impaired levels of consciousness.

Grand mal seizures involve rapid loss of consciousness with loss of muscle tone, tonic spasm, and jerks. The muscles become rigid for about 30 seconds during the tonic phase of the seizure and alternately contract and relax during the clonic phase, which lasts 30 to 60 seconds.

ALS for the BLS Provider

- Clear the area to protect the patient.
- Allow patient to stop seizing before attempting to provide care.
- Provide high-concentration oxygen via nonrebreathing mask and maintain airway.
- Prepare IV administration supplies.
- Prepare blood glucose testing equipment.
- Monitor oxygen saturation and end-tidal CO_2.

Key Questions

- How long did the seizure last?
- When was the last time the patient experienced a seizure?
- Have there been any changes in medication?
- Is the patient compliant in taking prescribed medications?
- When was the last medication-level blood work done?

- Is this the same type of seizure as those experienced in the past?
- Did the patient regain consciousness between seizures?
- What was going on during the seizure? Collect this information from bystanders.
- What is the patient's mental status (AVPU)?

Other Considerations

- Hypoglycemia
- Hypoxia
- Electrolyte imbalance
- Head injury, tumor
- Intoxication or poisoning

■ Stroke—CVA/TIA

Description A *stroke* is the sudden death of a portion of the brain cells due to a lack of oxygen. A stroke occurs when blood flow to the brain is impeded, resulting in abnormal function of the brain. It is caused by blockage or rupture of an artery to the brain.

Signs and Symptoms

- Sudden numbness or weakness, especially on one side of the body.
- Sudden confusion.

- Sudden vision problems in one or both eyes.
- Sudden difficulty walking, dizziness, loss of balance or coordination.
- Sudden, severe headache with no known cause.
- Sudden difficulty speaking or understanding speech.

ALS for the BLS Provider

- Apply oxygen immediately via nonrebreathing mask.
- Conduct a prehospital stroke scale evaluation to determine if patient fits criteria.
- Prep IV tubing, needles, and fluid for vascular access.
- Determine closest hospital that specializes in vascular access or TPA administration.
- Prepare for CPR or assisting in managing the patient's airway.
- Assist with application of the cardiac monitor.
- Ready possible medications (metoprolol [Lopressor], nitroglycerin).

Key Questions

- What was the exact time of onset? Within 3 hours?
- Stroke scale test?
- Did you evaluate pupils? Complete a motor/sensory exam?
- Is there any evidence of trauma?
- Obtain the following tests to rule out other issues:
  - Blood glucose
  - SpO_2
- Early hospital notification?

Other Considerations

- Hypoglycemia (obtain a blood glucose reading)
- Hypoxia (SpO_2)
- Infection (recent illness, stiff neck, fever)
- Brain tumor (history of cancer)
- Trauma (signs of recent or past trauma)
- Overdose/toxiciology (examine the scene for clues)

Medical

CINCINNATI STROKE SCALE

Screening Criteria	Yes	No
Ask the individual to smile.		
Does one side of the face droop or not move at all?	❏	❏
Ask the individual to raise both arms.		
Does one arm drift compared to the other?	❏	❏
Have the person say "You can't teach an old dog new tricks."		
Is the person slurring speech, using inappropriate words, or not speaking at all?	❏	❏

LOS ANGELES PREHOSPITAL STROKE SCALE

Screening Criteria	Yes	Unknown	No
1. Age > 45	❏	❏	❏
2. History of seizures or epilepsy absent	❏	❏	❏
3. Symptoms < 24 hours	❏	❏	❏
4. At baseline, patient is not wheelchair-bound or bedridden	❏	❏	❏
5. Blood glucose between 60 and 400	❏	❏	❏
6. Obvious asymmetry (right versus left) in any of the following three exam categories (must be unilateral):	❏	❏	❏

	Equal	Right Weak	Left Weak
Facial smile/grimace	❏	❏ Droop	❏ Droop
Grip	❏ ❏	❏ Weak Grip ❏ No Grip	❏ Weak Grip ❏ No Grip
Arm strength	❏ ❏	❏ Drifts Down ❏ Falls Rapidly	❏ Drifts Down ❏ Falls Rapidly

Interpretation: If criteria 1-6 are marked yes, the probability of a stroke is 97%.

■ Syncope

Description *Syncope* is the partial or complete loss of consciousness with interruption of awareness of one's self and surroundings. When the loss of consciousness is temporary and there is spontaneous recovery, it is referred to as *fainting.* Syncope is due to a temporary reduction in blood flow and therefore a shortage of oxygen to the brain. This leads to lightheadedness or a "blackout" episode (ie, a loss of consciousness).

Signs and Symptoms

Noncardiac Causes. Syncope is most commonly caused by conditions that do not directly involve the heart. These conditions include:

- Postural (orthostatic) hypotension, when blood pressure drops due to changing body position to a more vertical position after lying or sitting
- Dehydration causing a decrease in blood volume
- Blood pressure medications leading to low blood pressure
- Diseases of the nerves to the legs in older people (especially with diabetes or Parkinson's disease) when poor tone of the nerves of the legs draws blood into the legs from the brain
- High altitude

- Brain stroke or "near stroke" (transient ischemic attack)
- Migraine attack
- Fainting after certain situations (situational syncope), such as:
  - Blood drawing
  - Urinating (micturition syncope)
  - Defecating (defecation syncope)
  - Swallowing (swallowing syncope)
  - Coughing (cough syncope)

Cardiac Causes. Heart conditions that can cause syncope or fainting resulting in temporary loss of consciousness include:

- Abnormal heart rhythms (heart beating too fast or too slow)
- Abnormalities of the heart valves (aortic stenosis or pulmonic valve stenosis)
- High blood pressure in the arteries supplying the lungs (pulmonary artery hypertension)
- Tears in the aorta (aortic dissection)

ALS for the BLS Provider

- Provide high-concentration oxygen via nonrebreathing mask.
- Prepare blood glucose testing equipment.
- Attach 12-lead ECG monitoring equipment.
- Prepare IV supplies.

Other Considerations

- CVA
- Coronary syndrome
- Arrhythmia
- CHF
- Toxic exposure
- Pneumonia
- Pulmonary emboli
- Neurologic disease
- Hypoglycemia
- Dehydration
- Sepsis

Key Questions

- What position was the patient in prior to the event? Sitting, supine?
- Any symptoms with position changes?

Always rule on the side of cardiac cause until proven otherwise.

■ Trauma Assessment

- ■ Time of injury: When the injury occurred, not when you arrived at the scene.
- ■ Mechanism of injury: Estimated speed or cause.
- ■ Airway
  - • Open, position–jaw thrust, suction, insert airway
- ■ Breathing
  - • Respiratory rate and quality (spontaneous effort, work of breathing)
  - • Breath sounds
  - • Oxygen (bag-mask device)
  - • Signs of chest trauma
  - • Chest excursion and expansion
  - • Presence of flail segment
  - • Bony or air crepitus over chest or neck
  - • Complaint of shortness of breath
  - • Position of trachea
- ■ Circulation
  - • Major, uncontrollable bleeding
  - • Skin color, temperature, moisture
  - • Quality of pulses in all four extremities
  - • Capillary refill

Trauma

- Neurologic
  - Level of consciousness (GCS)
  - Ability to move all extremities
  - Posturing of extremities
  - Pupils
  - Recall of incident
  - Neck or back pain
  - Ear or nose drainage
  - Facial or head trauma
  - C-spine immobilization device, spinal precautions initiated
- Respiratory
  - Respiratory rate and quality
  - Type of oxygen
  - Breath sounds, repeat
  - Chest excursion and expansion
  - Complaint of shortness of breath
  - SpO_2
- Cardiovascular
  - Vital signs
  - Skin color, temperature, moisture
  - Capillary refill
  - Quality of pulses
- GI/GU
  - Signs of abdominal trauma
  - Quality of abdomen (soft/tender/rigid)

- Nausea, vomiting
- Pelvis stability, crepitus, pain
- Incontinence
- Musculoskeletal
  - Deformity, ecchymosis (bruising)
  - Swelling
  - Pulses, motor, sensory, distal to the injury site
  - Range of motion
  - Describe lacerations and abrasions

■ Thoracic Trauma

Flail Chest

Description Flail chest occurs when two or more adjacent ribs are fractured in more than one place.

Signs and Symptoms

- Paradoxical chest movement
- Intense pain
- Progressive shortness of breath or pain with chest wall movement

Trauma

ALS for the BLS Provider

- Stabilize flail segment.
- Provide oxygen and ventilation support.
- Support ALS with pain management, position of comfort, splinting, preparation of equipment, and repeat assessments.

Other Considerations

- Pneumothorax
- Rib fracture
- Aortic dissection

Key Questions

- Were the mechanics or force enough to cause pulmonary contusion?
- Repeated evaluation of lung sounds to check for pneumothorax?

Pulmonary Contusion

Description Pulmonary contusion involves bruised lung tissue and impaired gas exchange. It may present as respiratory failure. Look at respiratory status, work of breathing, and SpO$_2$.

Signs and Symptoms

- May present as respiratory failure
- Usually associated with major chest trauma
- Impaired respiratory function
- Increased work of breathing, difficulty breathing

- Chest pain
- Decreased SpO_2 despite aggressive airway and breathing efforts

ALS for the BLS Provider
- Support ventilation and oxygenation.
- May need to use bag-mask device.

Other Considerations
- Serious chest trauma
- Myocardial infarction
- Blunt cardiac injury
- Aortic injury

Key Questions
- Speed of accident? Was a restraint used?
- Signs of pneumothorax or tension pneumothorax?
- Signs of shock?

Pneumothorax

Description Pneumothorax is an accumulation of air or gas in the pleural cavity that occurs as a result of disease or injury. Sometimes induced to collapse the lung.

A *tension pneumothorax* is a medical emergency, because air accumulates in the pleural space with each breath. The continued increase in intrathoracic pressure results in

Trauma

massive shifts of the mediastinum away from the affected lung, compressing intrathoracic vessels.

If a pneumothorax occurs suddenly or for no known reason, it is called a *spontaneous pneumothorax.* This condition most often strikes tall, thin men ages 20 to 40.

Signs and Symptoms

- Simple pneumothorax
  - Caused by blunt or penetrating trauma
  - Breath sounds decreased or absent
  - Mild to moderate respiratory distress
- Tension pneumothorax
  - Breath sounds decreased or absent
  - Marked respiratory distress
  - Severe increase in work of breathing
  - Distended neck veins
  - Hemodynamic compromise

ALS for the BLS Provider

- Tension pneumothorax is life threatening. Prevent progression from simple to tension pneumothorax.
- Support ventilation and oxygenation.
- Assist with preparation of needle decompression.

Other Considerations

- Various other chest trauma
- Myocardial infarction
- COPD

Key Questions

- What are the breath sounds? Are they absent on one side?
- What do the neck veins look like?
- Is there a sucking chest wound?

Open Pneumothorax

Description An open pneumothorax is a penetrating trauma that results in a "sucking" chest wound. It is usually a large wound marked by respiratory distress. There is a free exchange between the exterior air and the pleural space either via the lung or through the chest wall, as through an open wound.

Signs and Symptoms

- Usually a large wound
- Marked respiratory distress

ALS for the BLS Provider

- Support ventilation and oxygenation.
- Clear and maintain the airway.
- Rapidly seal the open wound with a sterile occlusive dressing.

Trauma

ALS for the BLS Provider, cont.

- Continue to reassess to be sure a tension pneumothorax does not develop. Any patient with a penetrating chest wound must be watched closely at all times because tension pneumothorax may develop.
- Release one side on expiration, so the air can escape while the lung reinflates.

Other Considerations

- Myocardial infarction
- COPD
- CHF

Key Questions

- Any increased difficulty breathing?
- Taking a breath in or out when injury occurred?

Pericardial Tamponade

Description Pericardial tamponade occurs when blood or fluid collects in the pericardial sac. It is often seen with penetrating trauma.

Signs and Symptoms

- Faint heart sounds
- Weak pulse
- Low blood pressure
- Jugular vein distention

- Support ventilation and oxygenation.
- Arrange for rapid transport.
- Alert emergency department early.
- Do not delay transport waiting for ALS to arrive.

■ Traumatic Brain Injury

Description

- **Concussion/closed head injury.** Abnormal neurologic function due to trauma to the head.
- **Skull fractures.** Can be associated with traumatic brain injury.
- **Linear fractures.** Cannot be seen or palpated in the field.
- **Basilar fracture.** Can be associated with leakage of cerebrospinal fluid from the nose/ears. Raccoon eyes or Battle's sign may take hours to develop; do not rule out a fracture if not present on scene.
- **Depressed fracture.** Deformity noted on palpation.
- **Open fracture.** Cerebrospinal fluid and bleeding usually present, along with brain matter.

Trauma

Signs and Symptoms

- Abnormal neurologic function
- Possible loss of consciousness, disorientation
- Repetitive questions or statements
- Headache
- Vomiting

ALS for the BLS Provider

- Provide high-concentration oxygen via nonrebreathing mask.
- Provide C-spine immobilization.
- Prepare IV administration supplies.
- Prepare suction equipment.
- Prepare pulse oximetry monitoring equipment.

Key Questions

- Time of injury?
- Any loss of consciousness, even if brief?
- Recall of events, accident?
- Any loss of bladder function?
- Any blood or fluid noted in nose/ears (cerebrospinal fluid)?
- Repeated GCS exams? Neurologic exam should be repeatable by another person.
- Preventing secondary brain injury (avoiding hypoxia or hypotension)?

- If GCS is less than 9, do you need an advanced airway?
- Any past medical history that may affect level of consciousness?
- Check blood glucose (if local protocol allows).

Other Considerations

- Hypoglycemia
- Hypoxia
- Central nervous system event
- Myocardial infarction prior to trauma
- Sepsis/infection

■ Intracranial Hematomas

Description All the following types of hematomas can lead to intracranial hypertension and brain herniation:

- **Epidural.** Usually associated with temporal/parietal skull fractures, generally caused by arterial bleeding. Classically presents with a brief loss of consciousness after the injury, then a period of consciousness, and finally unresponsiveness.
- **Subdural.** Usually occurs over time from venous bleeding; slower progression.
- **Intracerebral.** Cerebral contusion, may expand over time.

Trauma

Signs and Symptoms

- Severe headache (*worst of their life*)
- Nausea and vomiting
- Altered mental status
- Hemiparesis
- Difficulty swallowing
- Visual field disturbance
- Coma
- Changes in respiratory pattern

ALS for the BLS Provider

- Prevent hypoxia and hypotension, which increase mortality rate.
- Maintain C-spine precautions.
- Establish an airway (be prepared for vomiting; prepare suction equipment).
- Support ventilation and oxygenation.
- Control any bleeding.
- Assess baseline mental status.
- Elevate head of stretcher/backboard to decrease intracranial pressure.
- If available, monitor ET_{CO_2} (30 to 35 mm Hg).
- Prevent hyperventilation unless there are signs of herniation.
- Think about appropriate destination for transport or intubation if GCS is less than 9.

Key Questions

- Any loss of consciousness?
- Repeated GCS exams?
- Any substance abuse? Does patient's medical history include dementia or other medical conditions affecting mentation?
- What is the baseline level of consciousness?

■ Spinal Trauma

Description Injury to the spinal tract results in same-side paralysis or loss of sensation of light touch, awareness of the body's position, and vibration. The sympathetic nervous system fibers exit from the spinal cord between C7 and L1. Neurogenic shock is characterized by severe autonomic dysfunction, resulting in hypotension, relative bradycardia, peripheral vasodilation, and hypothermia.

Signs and Symptoms

- Weakness, paralysis, pain, or numbness (may occur from impact or later from movement)
- Edema
- Ischemia
- Priapism

Trauma

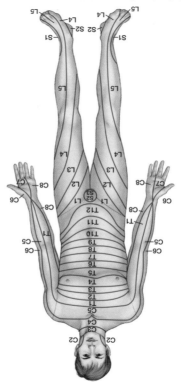

Spinal regions and dermatome areas

- Assess dermatomes to identify injury location. The principal dermatome levels are as follows:
  - C1/C2: Loss of ability to breathe
  - C4: Loss of diaphragm function, intercostal muscles
  - C5: Clavicles
  - C5-7: Lateral upper limbs
  - C8-T1: Medial upper limbs
  - C6: Thumb
  - C6-8: Hand
  - C8: Ring and little fingers
  - T4: Nipple level
  - T7: Xiphoid/epigastrium
  - T10: Umbilicus level
  - T12: Inguinal/groin area

■ Burns

Description Consider the type of burn (thermal, chemical, radiation) and the burn's location during early burn management. Once it has been determined that the burn is a thermal burn, add the following to the description: contact (with source name), scald (with fluid or gas type), heat, and flame. Systemic injury, duration, intentional versus accidental, and location of the burn must all be considered during the critical early burn period.

Trauma

Signs and Symptoms

- First-degree (superficial) burns involve only the epidermis:
  - Tissue blanches with pressure.
  - Tissue is erythematous (red) and often painful.
  - Tissue damage is minimal.
  - Sunburn is a classic example of this type of burn.
- Second-degree (partial-thickness) burns:
  - Epidermis and portions of the dermis are involved.
  - Sweat glands and hair follicles are often involved.
  - The burned area characteristically has blisters and is very painful.
  - If deep second-degree burns are not cared for properly, edema, which accompanies the injury, and decreased blood flow in the tissue can result in conversion to a full-thickness burn.
- Third-degree (full-thickness) burns:
  - Characterized by charring of skin or a translucent white color, with coagulated vessels visible below.
  - The area is insensate, but the patient complains of pain, which is usually a result of surrounding second-degree burns.

- Because all of the skin tissue and structures are destroyed, healing is very slow. Third-degree burns are often associated with extensive scarring, because epithelial cells from the skin appendages are not present to repopulate the area.
- Major burns:
  - All burns complicated by involvement of the respiratory tract:
    - Facial burns, singed or absent facial hair, hoarseness, stridor, soot in airway
  - Second- /third-degree burns of the face, hands, feet, or genitalia
  - Full-thickness burns of more than 10% body surface area
  - Partial-thickness burns of more than 30% body surface area
  - Burns complicated by trauma
  - Burns complicated by extensive past medical history
  - Comorbidities:
    - Age older than 55
    - Children younger than age 5 with full- or partial-thickness burns over more than 20% body surface area
    - Circumferential burns

Trauma

ALS for the BLS Provider

- Stop the burning process.
- Remove all clothing and jewelry.
- Provide high-concentration oxygen.
- Prepare intubation equipment.
- Provide early aggressive airway intervention before laryngeal edema.
- Consider aeromedical evacuation.

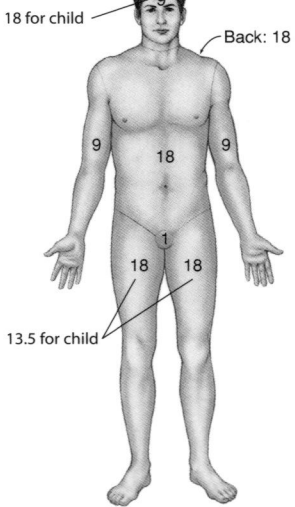

18 for child

Back: 18

9   18   9

1

18   18

13.5 for child

Rule of nines

This is the standard formula used for fluid replacement for burn patients:

$$4 \text{ mL/kg} \times \%BSA \div 24$$

The first half is to be given over the first 8 hours.

The following example reflects a patient weighing 80 kg, with burns over 70% of his body:

$$4 \text{ mL} \times 80 \text{ kg} \times 70\% \text{ BSA} \div 24$$
$$22400 \div 24 = 934 \text{ mL}$$
$$467 \text{ mL over 8 hours, 60 mL/h}$$

Key Questions

- Does assessment reveal inhalation injury?
- What percent of body surface area has been burned?
- Time of injury?
- Patient found in closed space or open area?
- Comorbid conditions (past medical history)?
- Signs of abuse, cigarette marks, glove or immersion burns?

Other Considerations

- Electrical injuries
- Chemical burns
- Carbon monoxide or cyanide poisoning

Trauma

ADULT INITIAL BURN RESUSCITATION (mL/HR)

Burn Size	Score (BSS)
Head	1
Arm/Hand	1
Ant. Torso	2
Back	2
Thigh/Leg	2

Total BSS	Weight (lbs) 88	110	132	154	176	198	220	242	264	286	308	330
	Weight (kg) 40	50	60	70	80	90	100	110	120	130	140	150
1	90	113	135	158	180	203	225	248	270	293	315	338
2	180	225	270	315	360	405	450	495	540	585	630	675
3	270	338	405	473	540	608	675	743	810	878	945	1013
4	360	450	540	630	720	810	900	990	1080	1170	1260	1350
5	450	563	675	788	900	1013	1125	1238	1350	1463	1575	1688
6	540	675	810	945	1080	1215	1350	1485	1620	1755	1890	2025
7	630	788	945	1103	1260	1418	1575	1733	1890	2048	2205	2363
8	720	900	1080	1260	1440	1620	1800	1980	2160	2340	2520	2700
9	810	1013	1215	1418	1620	1823	2025	2228	2430	2633	2835	3038
10	900	1125	1350	1575	1800	2025	2250	2475	2700	2925	3150	3375
11	990	1238	1485	1733	1980	2228	2475	2723	2970	3218	3465	3713

Courtesy of Christopher Lentz, MD, Strong Regional Burn Center

PEDIATRIC INITIAL BURN RESUSCITATION (mL/HR)

Burn Size Score (BSS)		Weight (kg)											
		(lbs) 13	20	26	33	40	46	53	59	66	73	79	86
		(kg) 6	9	12	15	18	21	24	27	30	33	36	39
Head (if < 30 kg 2)	1	**Total BSS**											
Arm/Hand	1	1	39	58	73	86	99	111	120	129	138	148	157	166
Chest/Abd	2	2	52	78	100	120	139	158	174	190	206	222	238	254
Back	2	3	66	98	127	153	180	205	228	251	273	296	319	342
Thigh/Leg (if < 30 kg 1.5)	2	4	79	119	154	187	220	252	282	311	341	370	400	429
		5	92	139	181	221	261	300	336	372	408	445	481	517
		6	106	159	208	255	301	347	390	433	476	519	562	605
		7	120	179	235	288	342	394	444	494	543	593	643	693
		8	133	200	262	322	382	441	498	554	611	667	724	780
		9	147	220	289	356	423	489	552	615	678	742	805	868
		10	160	240	316	390	463	536	606	676	746	816	886	956
		11	174	260	343	423	504	583	660	737	813	890	967	1044

Courtesy of Christopher Lentz, M[...]
Strong Regional Burn Center

Trauma

■ Chemical, Biologic, Radiologic, and Explosive Agents

There are four categories of terrorist agents:

- **Chemical agents.** Chemical agents are classified into six categories. U.S. military designations of chemical agents are listed in parentheses.

  - *Nerve agents.* Nerve agents disrupt nerve impulse transmission or cause peripheral nervous system effects. Exposure to even a small amount of a nerve agent can be fatal. [tabun (GA); sarin (GB/GB2); soman (GD); Cyclohexyl sarin (GF); nerve agent (VX/VX2); Soviet nerve agent (VR)]

  - *Blister agents (vesicants).* These agents are also known as *mustard* due to their characteristic smell. [Levinstein mustard (H); Lewisite (L); distilled mustard (HD/HS); ethyldichloroarsine (ED); methyldichloroarsine (MD); mustard T mixture (HT); nitrogen mustard (HN); mustard lewisite mixture (HL); phenyldichloroarsine (PD); phosgene oxime (CX)]

- *Blood agents*. Blood agents interfere with the ability of the blood to transport oxygen and result in asphyxiation. [hydrogen cyanide (AC); arsine (SA); cyanogen chloride (CK)]

- *Choking agents*. Choking agents stress the respiratory tract. Severe distress causes edema (fluid in the lungs), which can result in asphyxiation resembling drowning. [chlorine (CL); chloropicrin (PS); diphosgene (DP); phosgene (CG)]

- *Irritating agents*. Irritating agents, also known as *riot-control agents* or *tear gas*, are designed to incapacitate. [tear gas (CS); mace (CN); pepper spray (OC); tear gas (CR); vomiting agents (DA/DC/DM)]

- *Incapacitating agents*. Incapacitating agents cause hallucinations, confusion, and motor coordination problems. They also cause central and peripheral nervous system dysfunctions. [3-quinuclidinyl benzilate (BZ); Agent 15; lysergic acid diethylamide (LSD)]

- **Biologic Agents.** Biologic agents can be disseminated through food and water supply systems, direct contact with materials, or aerosolization. Biologic agents are classified into three general categories:

  - *Bacterial agents.* Bacterial agents are forms of bacteria. [*Bacillus anthracis* (anthrax); *Yersinia pestis* (plague); *Francisella tularensis* (tularemia); *Vibrio cholerae* (cholera); some rickettsial agents, such as *Coxiella burnetii* (Q fever), behave as bacterial agents]

  - *Viral agents.* Viral agents are forms of viruses. [viral hemorrhagic fever agents: Ebola, Venezuelan equine encephalitis (VEE); variola (smallpox)]

  - *Toxins.* Toxins are poisonous metabolites from fungi, plants, or bacteria. [castor bean toxin (ricin); botulinum toxin (botulism); staphylococcal enterotoxin *B* (SEB); mycotoxins (aflatoxins)]

- **Radiologic/nuclear agents.** Radiologic and nuclear incidents involve the use, threatened use, or threatened detonation of a nuclear device or a standard explosive incorporating nuclear materials (a radiologic dispersal device) or the distribution of radioactive materials.

The three primary types of radioactive energy are:

- *Alpha particles*. Alpha particles are heavy, highly charged particles that travel a few inches in the air. They can be stopped by paper.

- *Beta particles*. Beta particles are smaller, faster particles that travel a few millimeters through skin, but generally do not penetrate vital organs.

- *Gamma radiation*. Gamma radiation is electromagnetic radiation. It travels great distances and can penetrate most materials. Gamma radiation can attack tissues and organs.

- **Explosive/incendiary agents.** Explosive agents produce an extremely rapid release of gas under pressure, along with heat and fragmentation. Bombings, including the use of improvised devices, are the most common type of terrorist incident. FBI statistics identify that bombs nearly always work as designed. An incendiary device is a chemical, electrical, or mechanical device used to initiate combustion. The purpose of an incendiary agent is to set fire to other materials or structures. Devices generally contain a fuse, a container body, and an incendiary material.

■ Recognizing an Incident as Terrorism

You should be aware of the categories of agents and signs that may indicate a terrorist event in your jurisdiction. The following signs and symptoms may indicate that a terrorist event has occurred:

- Patients are unconscious with minimal or no trauma.
- Patients exhibit SLUDGEM signs/ symptoms:

  S Salivation (drooling)

  L Lacrimation (tearing)

  U Urination

  D Defecation, diarrhea

  G GI upset (cramps)

E Emesis (vomiting)

M Muscle twitching

- Patients are having difficulty breathing.
- Patients exhibit blistering, reddening, discoloration, or irritation of the skin.
- Multiple patients have the same signs and symptoms.

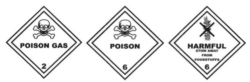

Placards and labels associated with chemical containers
Source: © Pedro Nogueira / Shutter Stock, Inc.

■ Specific Indicators of Chemical Agents

SYMPTOMS OF EXPOSURE: NERVE AGENTS

Agent
• GA: Tabun   • GF: Cyclohexyl sarin

- GA: Tabun
- GB: Sarin
- GB2: Sarin
- GD (VR-55): Soman

- GF: Cyclohexyl sarin
- VX: Nerve agent
- VX2: Nerve agent
- VR: Nerve agent (produced by the former Soviet Union)

Characteristics

- Attack the nervous system and disrupt nerve impulses.
- Can enter body through inhalation or through the skin.
- Tabun is primarily an inhalation hazard, whereas other agents are both inhalation and skin absorption/ingestion hazards.

- V agents are particularly potent inhalation and absorption/ingestion hazards due to their persistence.
- Rapid rate of action.
- Are semi-persistent (< 12 hours), though V agents are persistent (> 12 hours)

Exposure Symptoms

- Pinpoint pupils, blurred vision, pain aggravated by sunlight
- Runny nose and reports of unusual odors or tastes
- Drooling
- Coughing and difficulty breathing
- Tightness in chest

- Muscle twitching, jerking, excessive sweating
- Nausea, vomiting, diarrhea, involuntary defecation and urination
- Convulsions
- Coma
- Death

SYMPTOMS OF EXPOSURE: NERVE AGENTS (cont.)

Odors

- Tabun (GA): fruity when impure
- Sarin (GB): fruity when impure
- Soman (GD): none or camphor (mothballs)
- VX: none or sulfur

First Aid

- Use auto-injector immediately.
- Remove from area and treat symptomatically (atropine and 2-PAM chloride or H1-6).
- Soman can only be treated with H1-6.
- Pretreatment (carbamates) in low doses is effective and should be used in conjunction with auto-injectors.
- Diazepam is also used as a pretreatment and is most effective if administered 2 hours before exposure.

Note: Persistence is a measure of the duration for which the chemical agent is effective. A persistent agent retains its casualty-producing effects for an extended period of time, usually several days. A persistent agent usually has a low evaporation rate and is heavier than air.

SYMPTOMS OF EXPOSURE: BLISTER
AGENTS (VESICANTS)

Agent

- H: Mustard
- HD: (HS) Distilled mustard [less concentrated HD is known as Yperite (HS).]
- HL: Mustard–Lewisite mixture

- HN: Nitrogen mustard
- HT: Mustard T mixture
- L: Lewisite
- MD: Methyldichloroarsine
- CX: Phosgene oxime

Characteristics

- Attack skin and can also be inhaled.
- Absorbed rapidly into skin.
- Persistent (> 12 hours).

- Mustard has an asymptomatic latency period, whereas Lewisite causes immediate pain.

Exposure Symptoms

- Itching of eyes; tearing, swelling, and spasms of eyelids
- Nausea, vomiting, abdominal pain, blood-stained vomit and diarrhea
- Hoarseness or hacking cough, profusely runny nose, severe cough, shortness of breath
- Initial redness of skin, followed by blisters

- Skin effect varies with agent. Within 1 to 2 hours, mild itching followed by redness, pain, and fluid-filled blisters. Effects are enhanced in moist areas of groin and armpits.
- Mustard (H): No immediate effect.
- Lewisite (L): Immediate pain.

Odors

- Mustard gas (H): Garlic or onions. These agents are known as "mustard" due to their characteristic smell.

- Lewisite (L): Geraniums.
- Phosgene oxime: Irritating or peppery pungent odor

First Aid

- Decontaminate with large amounts of water.
- Remove clothing.

- Support airway.
- Treat symptomatically.

SYMPTOMS OF EXPOSURE: BLOOD AGENTS

Agent

- AC: Hydrogen cyanide
- CK: Cyanogen chloride
- SA: Arsine

Characteristics

- Attacks circulatory system.
- Gases stored in cylinders (under pressure, they are liquids).
- Blood agents are nonpersistent (lasting minutes to a few hours).
- Rate of action is rapid.

Exposure Symptoms

- Cherry red skin and lips
- Rapid breathing
- Dizziness, nausea
- Dilated pupils
- Excessive salivation
- Gastrointestinal hemorrhage
- Pulmonary edema
- Respiratory arrest
- Immediate onset of symptoms
- Loss of consciousness
- Convulsions
- Apnea
- Headache
- Respiratory distress (coughing and choking)
- Severe eye irritation
- Vertigo and headaches

SYMPTOMS OF EXPOSURE: BLOOD AGENTS (cont.)

Odors

- Hydrogen cyanide (AC): Bitter almonds or peaches
- Cyanogen chloride (CK): Bitter almonds
- Arsine (SA): Garlic

First Aid

- Rapid oxygen administration.
- Remove from area.
- Assist ventilation.
- Treat symptomatically.
- SA and CK may cause delayed pulmonary edemas.

SYMPTOMS OF EXPOSURE: CHOKING AGENTS

Agent

- CG: Phosgene (Collongite)
- DP: Diphosgene (Superpalite)
- CL: Chlorine
- PS: Chloropicrin

Characteristics

- Attack respiratory tract.
- Nonpersistent (minutes to a few hours).
- Vapors may hang in low areas.

Exposure Symptoms

- Coughing, nausea, choking, vomiting
- Irritated eyes, nose, throat
- Shortness of breath
- Pulmonary edema
- Frothy secretions

Odors

- Phosgene (CG): Newly mown hay or green corn.
- Chlorine (CL): Pool water
- Diphosgene (DP): Cut grass or green corn

First Aid

- Remove from area.
- Remove contaminated clothing.
- Ensure forced rest in a semi-upright position.
- Assist ventilation and respiration.
- Oxygen may be required for respiratory distress.

SYMPTOMS OF EXPOSURE: IRRITATING AGENTS

Agent

- OC: Pepper spray
- CA: Bromobenzylcyanide[1]
- CN (CNC, CNS, CNB)[2]: Mace
- CS: Tear gas
- CR: Tear gas

- DA: Diphenylchloroarsine (vomiting agent)
- DC: Diphenylcyanoarsine[3] (vomiting agent)
- DM: Adamsite (vomiting agent)

Characteristics

- Designed to incapacitate.
- Many are commercially available.
- Nonlethal; however, can result in asphyxiation under certain circumstances.

- Rapid rate of action.
- Tear gas (CS and CR) is persistent on porous surfaces.

Exposure Symptoms

- Burning or irritation of the eyes, throat, and skin in moist areas.
- Respiratory system distress, coughing, choking, difficulty breathing.

- High concentrations may lead to nausea or vomiting.

Weapons of
Mass Destruction

Odor

• CN: Apple blossoms	• CS/OC: Pepper-like odor

First Aid

• Remove from area.	• Remove contaminated clothing.
• Support respirations.	• Wash skin with soap and water.
• Treat symptomatically.	

[1] May be known as CAMITE.

[2] Chloroacetophenone (CN) is sometimes distributed in chloroform (CNC) with cloropicrin in chloroform (CNS) or in benzene and carbon tetrachloride (CNB). CNC has an odor of chloroform. CNS has an odor of fly paper. CNB has an odor of benzene.

[3] Diphenylcycinoarsine (DP) may be known as STERNITE; it is sometimes used in conjunction with Sarin (GB).

■ Toxic Exposure

Description A hazardous material is a substance (natural, chemical, biologic, radiologic, or explosive) that can be inhaled, ingested, absorbed, or injected and that can be considered harmful to one's health. Responders should use appropriate personal protective equipment (PPE) and use the principles of time, distance, and shielding.

Signs and Symptoms

- Fever
- Flulike symptoms
- Chills
- Headache
- Cough, difficulty breathing
- Local sores/lesions

Key Considerations

- Response to a target hazard or target event
- Disruptions to critical systems (such as transportation or utilities)
- Receipt of a threat
- An explosion, particularly if there is a debris field
- A secondary attack/explosion
- Multiple nontrauma-related patients
- Responders who are patients

- Hazardous substances involved in the incident
- Severe structural damage without an obvious cause
- Dead animals or vegetation
- Unusual odors, color of smoke, or vapor clouds

Affirmative answers to the following questions may indicate the use of a terroristic agent:

- Any clustering of symptoms or symptoms unusual for age of patients?
- Impact to humans, plants, and animals?
- Any unusual clustering of patients' time and location?
- Is the release location inconsistent with chemical use?
- Are any SLUDGEM symptoms apparent?
- Are patients exhibiting shortness of breath, chest pain, headache, suicidal/ homicidal behavior?
- Are patients exhibiting altered mental status, vomiting, cough, eye irritation, or seizures?

In the case of a potential terrorist attack, take the following precautions:

- Maintain patients' airways.
- Decontaminate area of exposure.

- Notify the closest hospitals as soon as possible.
- Consider a secondary device.
- Consider an antidote, if available (Mark 1 kit).

ALS for the BLS Provider

- Apply oxygen via nonrebreathing mask.
- Prepare IV supplies (two sets of tubing and preparation kits may be needed).
- Test blood glucose.
- Test SpO_2.
- Contact medical control.
- Contact poison control.

Key Questions

- Is the scene safe? Is appropriate personal protective equipment available?
- Activity at onset? Was onset of symptoms gradual or sudden?
- What type of behavior or symptoms?
- When did exposure occur (time, distance, shielding)?
- Is AMS present? If so, check blood glucose.
- Timing of the event (anniversary, holiday)?
- Are an unusual number of victims seeking care for skin, neurologic, respiratory, or GI symptoms?

■ Landing Zone Operations

Scene (landing zone) information only!

- The flight crew will obtain patient report when safely landed.
- One person is assigned to landing the aircraft safely, and that is that person's only responsibility.
- Aircraft will try to contact landing zone officer about 5 to 10 minutes out.
- Landing zone officer may need to be on apparatus radio; portable may not transmit.
- Focus all attention on managing communications, approach/departure, and landing site area.
- Landing zone
  - Proximity to the accident
  - 100' × 100'
  - Level surface
  - Clear of obstructions
  - Secured by landing zone officer
  - Approach and departure path clear of obstructions

■ Marking the Landing Zone

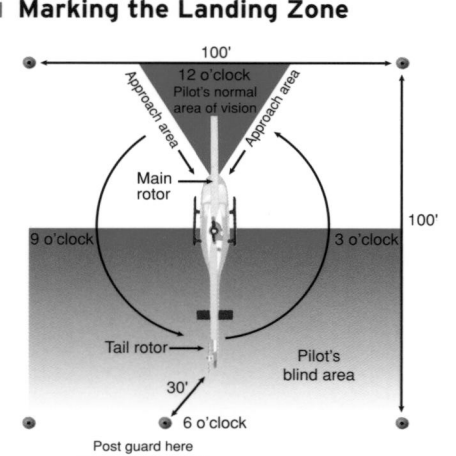

Landing zone markings

Daytime Markings

- Flares (caution)
- Cones
- Rescue vehicles
- Overhead lighting on rescue vehicles both for day and night

Nighttime Markings

- Flares (caution)
- Chemical light sticks

- Battery-powered flashlights (secured to ground)
- Headlights from two vehicles pointed at landing zone to form an X

Key Points

- Secure loose debris (car doors, trunk lids, stretchers, linens, baseball hats, etc.).
- Protect yourself. Wear turnout gear, goggles, and protective eye shields.
- Walk through landing zone.
- Secure nearby activities:
  - Moving traffic
  - Rescue activity
- Close apparatus and ambulance doors.
- Keep all spectators more than 200' from landing zone. Only those assigned to protect the aircraft are allowed within 100'.
- Always approach the aircraft from the nose.
- Never approach the aircraft unless directed by the flight crew or pilot.
- If asked to get equipment by flight crew in aircraft, never approach without getting the pilot's attention.
- Keep all personnel and others at least 50' away from the aircraft when running.

Operations

- A safety officer should be placed 30′ behind the tail rotor.
- *Never* approach the tail rotor of the aircraft!
- Let the flight crew come to you.
- The flight crew *does not* require assistance off-loading equipment.
- Keep apparatus and EMS vehicle doors and windows closed.
- Leave patient in ambulance. Carry nothing above the waist level.
- No smoking within 50′ of the aircraft.
- No sheets, blankets, or baseball hats near the aircraft.

Departure Information

- Limit communications to hazards only.
- Ensure that aircraft and tail rotor are clear of obstructions.
- Maintain visual contact with the aircraft until clear of landing zone.
- Maintain radio communications with the pilot until the aircraft is safely in forward flight.
- Immediately report any safety concerns to the pilot, again using short, simple commands.

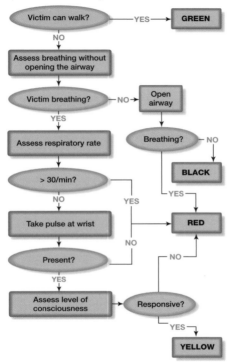

Priorities

- **P1**—Life-threatening illness or injury, ABC difficulties, decreased mental status. Treatment limited to opening the airway. Treatable injuries requiring rapid medical attention. Code RED.
- **P2**—Serious, but not life threatening, stable enough to wait a short while for medical treatment. Major, multiple fractures. Code YELLOW.
- **P3**—Walking wounded; minor injuries. Code GREEN.
- **P0**—Expectant, deceased, fatal injuries. Code BLACK.

■ Mass Casualty Incident (MCI)

- Assess dispatch information.
- Think about additional resources.
- Dispatch notification of closest hospital facilities (early walk-ins).
- Possible WMD signs?
- Is the scene safe to enter?
- Scene size? Provide quick description and number of victims in first report.
- Don command vest.
- Locate police and fire personnel (established unified command).

- Declare a mass casualty incident.
- Indicate/request the following:
  - Extent of the incident
  - Contained or ongoing incident
  - Command post location
  - Additional resources needed (ALS, BLS, physician to the scene)
  - Best routes of access
  - Staging area
  - Radio frequency priority
- Designate staging officer early to prevent traffic jam.
- Designate triage officer.
- Roll call of hospital(s) available.
- Designate treatment officer (if needed).
- Designate field hospital (if needed).
- Are specialized resources (UTSAR, HazMat, aeromedical, utility, bus, school/sheltering) needed?

■ HazMat Classifications

- Class 1: Explosives (six divisions)
  1.1–Mass explosion hazard
  1.2–Projectile hazard
  1.3–Minor blast/projectile/fire

1.4–Minor blast

1.5–Insensitive explosives

1.6–Very insensitive explosives

- Class 2: Gases (three divisions)

  2.1–Flammable

  2.2–Nonflammable compressed

  2.3–Poisonous

- Class 3: Flammable and Combustible Liquids and Gases

  - Flammable
    - Flash point below 141ºF
  - Combustible
    - Flash point 141º–200ºF

- Class 4: Flammable Solids

  4.1–Flammable solids

  4.2–Spontaneously combustible

  4.3–Dangerous when wet

- Class 5: Oxidizers and Organic Peroxides

  5.1–Oxidizers

  5.2–Organic peroxide

- Class 6: Poisons

  6.1–Material that is poisonous

  6.2–Infectious agents

- Class 7: Radioactive

- Class 8: Corrosives

- Class 9: Miscellaneous (ORM)
- ORM-D: Consumer Commodities

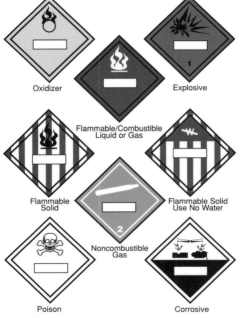

Oxidizer

Flammable/Combustible
Liquid or Gas

Explosive

Flammable
Solid

Noncombustible
Gas

Flammable Solid
Use No Water

Poison

Corrosive

HazMat placards

Operations

■ CPR Administration

CPR ADMINISTRATION

Adult (8 years and older) Child (1 to 8 years)	Infant (younger than 1 year)
Check for response Shake and shout	Tap foot
Call 9-1-1 As soon as possible after you find no response	After 2 minutes of CPR
Open the airway Head tilt–chin lift	Head tilt–chin lift (Caution: Do not hyperextend neck.)
Check for breathing Look, listen, and feel for no longer than 5 to 10 seconds. (If not breathing, give two breaths that make the chest rise over 1 to 1.5 seconds.)	Look, listen, and feel for no longer than 5 to 10 seconds. (If not breathing, give two breaths that make the chest rise over 1 to 1.5 seconds.)

Rescue breathing

12 breaths/min	20 breaths/min

Check for signs of circulation (No longer than 5 to 10 seconds)

Coughing, breathing, movement, turning blue. Check for carotid pulse.	Coughing, breathing, movement, turning blue. Check for brachial pulse.

Start CPR

Give cycles of 30 compressions to 2 breaths.	Give cycles of 30 compressions to 2 breaths.

Hand location

Center of chest, between nipples	Just below nipple line

Depth

1.5 to 2 inches	One third to one half chest diameter

Rate

100 per minute	100 per minute

Procedures

Adult (8 years and older) Child (1 to 8 years)	Infant (younger than 1 year) (cont.)
AED	
• Stop CPR and turn on AED.	• Stop CPR and turn on AED.
• Select proper size electrodes.	• Select proper size electrodes
• Apply pads.	• Apply pads.
• Analyze rhythm.	• Analyze rhythm.
• Clear victim to shock, if indicated.	• Clear victim to shock, if indicated.
Continue CPR	
Resume CPR immediately after delivery of shock.	Resume CPR immediately after delivery of shock.
Limit interruptions to chest compressions.	Limit interruptions to chest compressions.

■ Aspirin Administration

- Take BSI precautions.
- Ensure adequate ABCs.
- Administer high-concentration oxygen.
- Place patient in position of comfort.
- Obtain vital signs.

- If chest pain is present and is cardiac in nature, request ALS, if available.
- Check patient for allergies to aspirin:
  - If no allergies or recent GI bleeding, administer non-enteric chewable aspirin (160 to 325 mg).
- Provide rapid transport to a primary cardiac vascular specialty hospital. Request ALS intercept, if possible, or continue on. *Do not delay transport*.
- Provide ongoing assessment, recheck vital signs, repeat en route.
- Document medication administration on patient care report.

■ Blood Glucose Testing

- Take BSI precautions; wash your hands.
- Prepare the blood glucose meter and supplies.
- Make sure control matches strip.
- Cleanse the skin; do not use alcohol.
- Use lancet or device to perform a fingerstick. Use the sides of the fingertip pads; this results in less pain and less callus.
- Apply blood sample to strip.

Procedures

- Dispose of all sharps in appropriate biohazard container.
- Read blood glucose meter. Normal range is 70 to 120 mg/dL.
- If symptomatic and blood glucose is less than 80 mg/dL, review diabetic emergency section of local protocols. Contact ALS as soon as possible.

■ 12-Lead ECG Placement

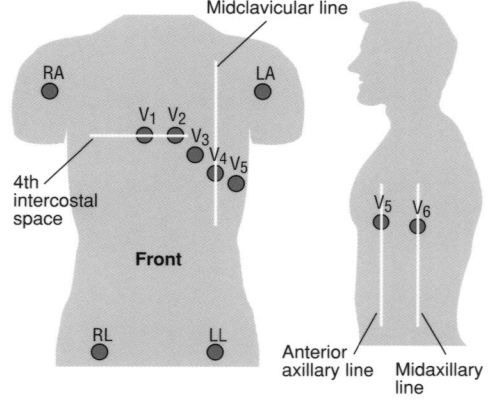

ECG placement

Prepare Patient's Skin

- Patients in cardiac distress situations can be diaphoretic (sweaty). The skin will need to be dried thoroughly so that the leads will stick to the patient's skin and transmit a good reading. Use alcohol to clean the skin if unable to stick electrodes.
- Remove any excess hair. Leads floating above the skin will not transmit accurate readings.

Place Electrodes on Skin

One lead goes on each limb: left shoulder, left leg, right shoulder, right leg.

- V_1–Fourth intercostal space to the right of the sternum
- V_2–Fourth intercostal space to the left of the sternum
- V_3–Directly between leads V_2 and V_4
- V_4–Fifth intercostal space at midclavicular line
- V_5–Beyond V_4 at left anterior axillary line
- V_6–Level with V_5 at left midaxillary line (directly under the midpoint of the armpit)

Procedures

■ Oral Glucose Administration

Indications

Glucose should be administered orally if patient presents with an altered mental status and has a known history of diabetes controlled by medication.

Contraindications

Oral glucose administration is contraindicated if the patient is unresponsive or unable to swallow.

Actions

Oral glucose administration increases blood glucose.

Side Effects

When given properly, no side effects result. If patient does not have a gag reflex, he or she may aspirate the glucose.

Dosage

- Adult: One tube
- Child: One tube (follow local protocol)

Suggested Steps for Administration

- Patient must be conscious and able to swallow.
- Consult medical direction for authorization.
- Administer glucose between the patient's cheek and gums.
- If a tongue depressor is used:

- Place glucose on bottom third of tongue depressor.
- Place tongue depressor between the patient's cheek and gums, with gel toward the cheek.
- Allow gel to dissolve or instruct patient to swallow it.

Consider other possible causes of altered mental status:

- Head trauma
- Seizures
- Poisoning
- Infection
- Hypoxia (decreased oxygen level)
- Hypothermia or hyperthermia
- Intoxication (other medical problems may still be present)

Epinephrine Auto-Injector

Indications

Patient must meet the following three criteria for use of an epinephrine auto-injector:

- Patient must exhibit symptoms of an allergic reaction (primarily those of a severe reaction, including respiratory

Procedures

distress and/or signs and symptoms of shock).

- Medication must be prescribed for this patient.
- Medical direction must authorize use for this patient.

Contraindications

None when used in a life-threatening situation.

Actions

Dilates the bronchioles; constricts blood vessels.

Side Effects

- Increased pulse rate
- Pallor
- Dizziness
- Chest pain
- Headache
- Nausea
- Vomiting
- Excitability, anxiousness

Dosage

- Adult: One adult auto-injector (0.3 mg)
- Child and infant: One infant/child auto-injector (0.15 mg)

Suggested Steps for Administration

- Obtain patient's prescribed auto-injector or BLS injector, if applicable.

- If able to see medication, do not use if discolored.
- Remove safety cap.
- If possible, remove clothing from injection site (can be administered through thin clothing, if necessary).
- If possible, wipe injection site with alcohol.
- Place tip of injector against the lateral portion of the patient's thigh midway between the waist and knee (can also inject in fleshy portion of patient's upper arm).
- Push firmly until injector activates.
- Hold injector in place 10 seconds or until medication is injected.
- Massage the site to enhance absorption.
- Dispose of auto-injector in proper biohazard container.

Additional Notes

- Take the auto-injector with the patient to the hospital.
- Medical direction may order a second dose.
- Some patients also carry oral antihistamines. If available, consult medical direction concerning their use.

Procedures

Common Signs and Symptoms of an Allergic Reaction

Respiratory

- Wheezing, stridor, or cough
- Tight feeling in the throat or chest
- Rapid breathing

Skin

- Itching
- Flushed (red) skin
- Hives
- Swelling (especially of the face, neck, tongue, hands, and/or feet)

Cardiac

- Increased pulse
- Decreased blood pressure

Other

- Runny nose
- Itchy, watery eyes
- Headache
- Nausea and/or vomiting
- Altered mental status

■ Nitroglycerin Administration

Indications

Patient must meet the following three criteria:

- Patient exhibits signs and symptoms of chest pain.
- Medication must be prescribed for this patient.
- Medical direction must authorize use for this patient.

Contraindications

- Hypotension or systolic blood pressure below 100 mm Hg (follow local protocol).
- Head injury
- Patient is an infant or child.
- Patient has already reached maximum prescribed dose for medication prior to EMT arrival.
- Patient is taking sildenafil (Viagra) or other erectile dysfunction medication. (Consult medical direction. Nitroglycerin may cause a serious drop in this patient's blood pressure.)

Actions

Dilates coronary arteries, increasing blood flow and oxygen supply to heart muscle; relaxes smooth muscle of blood vessel walls; decreases workload of heart.

Procedures

Side Effects

- Hypotension
- Headache
- Pulse rate changes

Dosage

- Adult: One dose, repeated in 3 to 5 minutes if:
  - No relief of pain, *and*
  - Blood pressure remains above 100 mm Hg systolic, *and*
  - Medical direction authorizes additional doses (*up to a maximum of three doses*).
- Child and infant: *Not for children or infants.*

Suggested Steps for Administration

- Patient's blood pressure must be above 100 mm Hg systolic.
- Check the expiration date of the medication. If nitroglycerin is older than 6 months, it may have lost its potency. (If the prescription is old, the EMT may ask if patient has a newer bottle.)
- Ask if the patient has already taken any, and, if so, how many were taken, when, and the effects of the medication on the patient.

If Medical Control Orders Administration

- Wear gloves. Nitroglycerin can be absorbed through the skin and can affect the EMT the same as it does the patient.
- Have patient lift tongue and place tablet or spray dose under tongue.
- If nitroglycerin is a tablet, advise patient to close his or her mouth and not to chew or swallow until the tablet dissolves and is absorbed.
- Recheck the patient's blood pressure within 2 minutes.

Additional Notes

- Continually monitor patient's blood pressure.
- If blood pressure drops or the patient feels faint, lay the patient down.
- Ask patient about pain relief.
- Ask patient whether the medication burned under the tongue or caused a headache.
- Seek medical direction before re-administering.
- If a patient who must be defibrillated is wearing a nitroglycerin patch, remove it before defibrillating.

Procedures

■ Metered-Dose Inhaler

Indications

Patient must meet all the following criteria:

- Patient must exhibit signs and symptoms of a respiratory emergency (wheezing may be heard when listening to breath sounds).
- Patient must have a prescribed inhaler.
- Medical direction must give authorization for use.

Contraindications

- Patient is unable to use device.
- Inhaler is not prescribed for the patient.
- Medical direction does not grant permission for use.
- Patient has already reached maximum prescribed dose for medication prior to EMT arrival.

Actions

Relaxes smooth muscles in the bronchial tubes, causing them to dilate, thus making breathing easier.

Side Effects

- Increased pulse rate
- Tremors
- Nervousness

Dosage

Adult and child: Maximum number of inhalations varies. Total number is based on orders from medical direction or orders from the patient's physician (consult with patient).

COMMON INHALER NAMES

Generic Name	Trade Name
Albuterol	Proventil, Ventolin
Bitolterolmesylate	Tornalate
Isoetharine	Bronkometer, Bronkosol
Metaproterenol	Alupent, Metaprel
Salmeterol xinofoate	Serevent

Suggested Steps for Administration

- Ask if the patient has already taken any doses and compare with prescribed dose.
- Ensure that the inhaler is at room temperature or warmer.
- Shake the inhaler vigorously for at least 30 seconds.
- If a spacer device is available, place it on the inhaler.
- Remove oxygen mask from the patient (an oxygen cannula can be left on).
- Have patient exhale deeply.

Procedures

- Tell the patient to put the mouthpiece in his or her mouth and make a seal with the lips.
- Instruct the patient to inhale slowly and deeply for more than 5 seconds and depress the patient's inhaler canister to deliver medication while the patient is inhaling.
- Have the patient hold his or her breath for as long as comfortably possible.
- Place the patient back on oxygen.

Additional Notes

- Medical direction may order additional doses.
- If an over-the-counter inhaler is present, the EMT will not likely assist the patient in using it.

Special Notes About Children With Asthma

- When experiencing asthma-related bronchospasms, children will often cough rather than wheeze.
- Look for retractions, use of accessory muscles (eg, neck, back, and abdominal muscles), and/or nasal flaring as indications of respiratory distress.

■ Intubation

Positioning is key to successful intubation! The goal is to align the three axes of the airway.

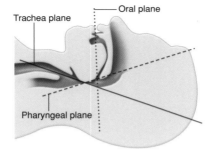

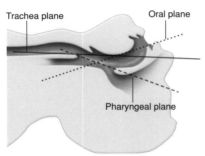

Three axes of the airway

- Apply towels
  - Under head for older patients
  - Under shoulders for younger patients

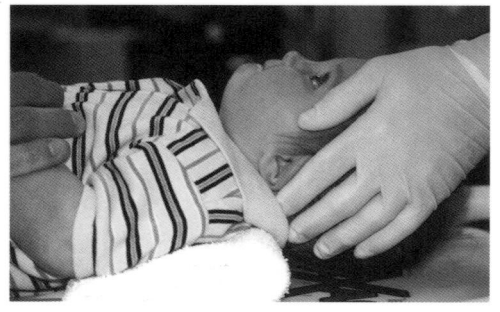

Use of a shoulder roll with an infant

- Apply gentle cricoid pressure during intubation.

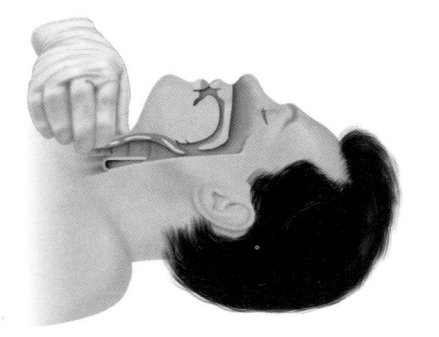

Cricoid pressure (Sellick maneuver)

LMA Sizing

LMA Size	Patient Size
1	Neonates/infants < 5 kg
1 ½	Infants 5 to 10 kg
2	Infants/children 10 to 20 kg
2 ½	Children 20 to 30 kg
3	Children/small adults 30 to 50 kg
4	Adults 50 to 70 kg
5	Large adult > 70 kg

Combitube

- Two sizes
  - Small (patients 4 to 5.5 feet tall)
  - Regular (patients over 5.5 feet tall)
- Not useful in most children
- Easy to place
- Contraindications
  - Gag reflex
  - Esophageal disease
  - Caustic ingestions
  - Foreign bodies/airway obstruction

Procedures

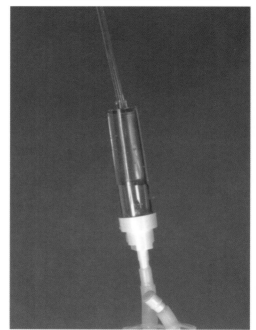

■ IV Setup

Spiking the Bag

Slide the spike into the IV bag port.

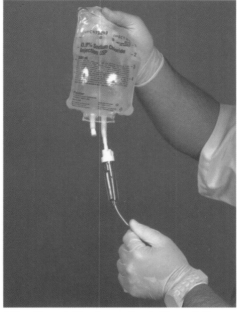

Allow the solution to run freely through the drip chamber and into the tubing to prime the line and flush the air out of the tubing. Let the fluid flow until air bubbles are removed from the line before turning the roller clamp wheel to stop the flow.

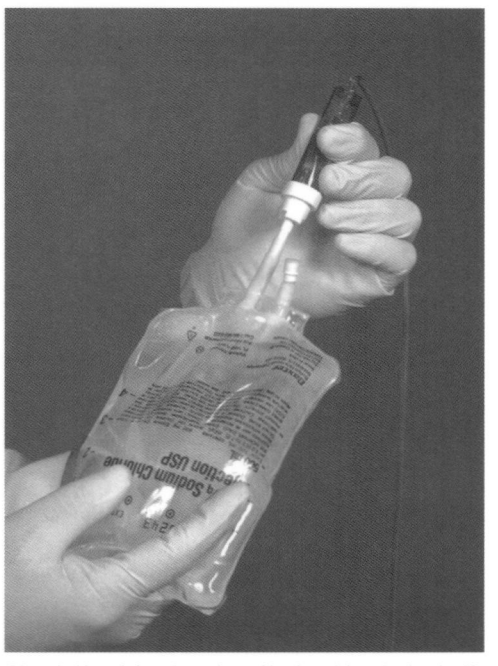

Check the drip chamber; it should only be half filled. Hang the bag in an appropriate location.

IV Therapy

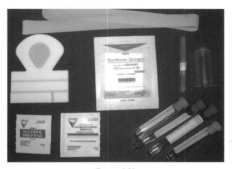

Prep kit

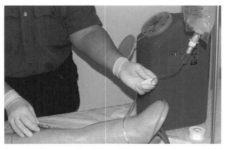

ALS will open the IV line to ensure that fluid is flowing and the IV is patent. Observe for any swelling or infiltration around the IV site.

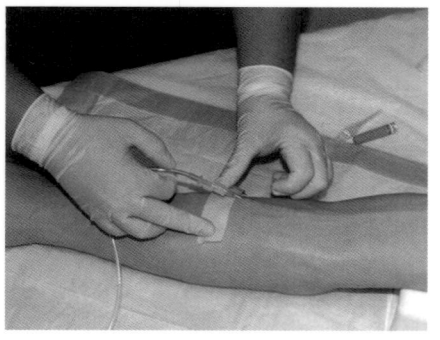

Help secure the catheter with tape or a commercial device.

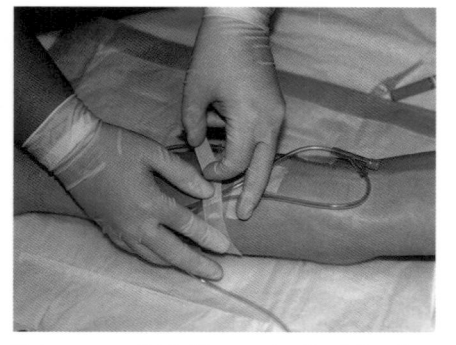

Help secure IV tubing and adjust the flow rate while monitoring the patient.

■ Intraosseous IV–Pediatric

Intraosseous IV is indicated for children younger than 8 years who are in shock, cardiac arrest, or unresponsive to verbal stimuli *and* unconscious or seriously ill. If one or two attempts at peripheral venipuncture have been unsuccessful within 90 seconds, ALS providers may use an intraosseous IV to administer fluids or drugs.

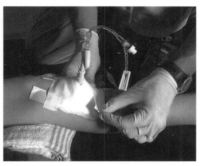

Help secure the needle with tape and support it with a bulky dressing. Secure the site with a splint.

■ ETco$_2$–Waveform Interpretation

Normal ETco$_2$ range is 35 to 45 mm Hg. The following three questions should be asked every time capnography is used:

Procedures

1. Is the ET tube in the trachea (rise and fall of detectable CO$_2$)?
2. What is the ETCO$_2$ value (height of the waveform)?
3. What is the shape of the waveform?

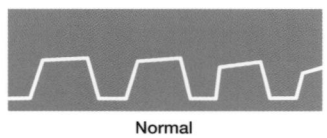

Normal

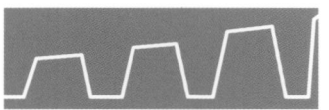

Hypoventilation

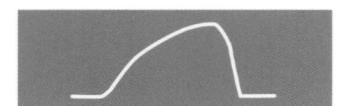

COPD/Asthma

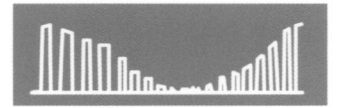

Cardiac Arrest

Normal, hypoventilation, COPD/asthma, cardiac arrest waveforms

ETT Dislodge

ETT dislodge waveform

■ Pulse Oximetry

PULSE OXIMETRY INTERVENTIONS

Range	EMS Interventions
Normal: 95-100%	None
Mild hypoxia: 91-94%	Administer O_2
Moderate hypoxia: 86-90%	Administer 100% O_2
Severe hypoxia: < 85%	100% O_2, ventilate

False low SpO_2 readings may be caused by the following:

- Poor peripheral circulation
- Hypothermia

False high SpO_2 readings may be caused by:

- Anemia
- Carbon monoxide poisoning

When in doubt, give oxygen!

Procedures

The following are common medications used for various conditions. Trade names are identified with capital letters. Generic equivalents are in parentheses.

■ Asthma

ACCOLATE (zafirlukast)

AEROBID (flunisolide)

AEROLATE (theophylline)

ALUPENT (metaproterenol)

AZMACORT (triamcinolone)

BECLOVENT (beclomethasone)

BRETHINE (terbutaline)

DILOR (dyphylline)

FLOVENT (fluticasone)

INTAL (cromolyn)

PULMICORT (budesonide)

RESPBID (theophylline)

SEREVENT (salmeterol)

SLO-BID (theophylline)

THEODUR (theophylline)

VENTOLIN (albuterol)

ZYRTEC (cetirizine)

■ Blood Thinners (Anticoagulants)

ACUPRIN 81 (aspirin, Ecotrin)

Aspirin (acetylsalicylic acid)

COUMADIN (warfarin)

PLAVIX (clopidogrel bisulfate)

TICLID (ticlopidine)

■ Cardiac Conditions

ADALAT (nifedipine)

BETAPACE (sotalol)

CALAN (verapamil)

CARDENE (nicardipine)

CARDIZEM (dilitiazem)

COREG (carvedilol)

COVERA (verapamil)

INDERAL (propranolol)

ISMO (isosorbide mononitrate)

ISOPTIN (verapamil)

ISORDIL (isosorbide dinatrate)

LANOXIN (digoxin, digitoxin)

LOPRESSOR (metoprolol)

NITRO-BID, NITRO-DUR (nitroglycerin)

NORMODYNE (labetalol)

QUINIDEX (quinidine)

TENORMIN (atenolol)
TIAZAC (dilitiazem)
TIMOLOL (blocadren)
VASCOR (bepridil)
ZIAC (bisoprolol)

■ CHF Diuretics

ACCUPRIL (quinapril)–ACE inhibitor
ALDACTONE (spironolactone)
APRESOLINE (hydralazine, HCTZ)
BUMEX (bumetanide)
CAPOTEN (captopril)–ACE inhibitor
COREG (carvedilol)
CRYSTODIGIN (digitoxin)
DYAZIDE (HCTZ, triameterene)
HCTZ (hydrochlorothiazide)
LANOXIN (digoxin)
LASIX (furosemide)
LOTENSIN (benazepril)
MIDAMOR (amiloride)
MODURETIC (amiloride, HCTZ)
PRINIVIL (lisinopril)
VASOTEC (enalapril)
ZAROXOLYN (metolazone)

ZESTERIL (lisinopril)
ZESTORETIC (lisinopril)

■ COPD

AEROLATE (theophylline)
ALUPENT (metaproterenol)
ATROVENT (metaproterenol)
BECLOVENT (beclomethasone)
PROVENTIL (albuterol)
RESPBID (theophylline)
SEREVENT (salmeterol)
SLO-BID (theophylline)
THEODUR (theophylline)
UNIPHYL (theophylline)
VENTOLIN (albuterol)

■ Dementia (Alzheimer's, Parkinson's)

ARICEPT (donepezil)
ARTANE (trihexyphenidyl)
ATAMET, SINEMET (carbidopa, levodopa)
COGENTIN (benztropine)
PARLODEL (bromocriptine)

PERMAX (pergolide)
SYMMETREL (amantadine)

■ **Diabetes**

ACTOS (pioglitizone)
AMARYL (glimepiride)
AVANDIA (rosiglitazone)
DIABETA (glyburide)
DIABINESE (chlorproamide)
GLUCOPHAGE (metformin)
GLUCOTROL (glipizide, glynase)
GLUCOVANCE (combination therapy of
    metformin and glyburide)
HUMULIN N, HUMULIN R (insulin)
LANTUS (insulin)
MICRONASE (glyburide)
MIGLITOL (glyset)
NATEGLINIDE (Starlix)
NOVOLIN, NOVOLOG (insulin)
NPH (insulin)
PRANDIN (repaglinide)
PRECOSE (acarbose)

■ GI Illness

AMPHOGEL (aluminum hydroxide)

ANTIVERT, BONINE (meclizine)—antinausea, vertigo

BELLADENAL (belladonna)—irritable bowel

CARAFATE (sucralfate)—anti-ulcer

COLACE, PERI-COLACE (docusate)—stool softener

COMPAZINE (prochlorperazine)—antinausea

DONNAGEL (pectin)

LOMOTIL (diphenoxylate, atropine)—antidiarrheal

PHENERGAN (promethazine)—antinausea

PRILOSEC (omeprazole)—ulcer, gastric secretions

REGLAN (metoclopramide)—heartburn, ulcers

SENOKOT (senna extract)—laxative

TIGAN (trimethobenzamide)—antinausea

TRANSDERM-SCOP (scopolamine)—antinausea, motion sickness

ZANTAC (ranitidine)—ulcers

■ Hypertension

ACCUPRIL (quinapril)—ACE inhibitor

ALDOMET (methyldopa)

ALTACE (ramipril)

APRESOLINE (hydralazine)

BETAPACE (sotalol)

CAPOTEN (captopril)–ACE inhibitor

CARDENE (nicardipine)

CARDIZEM (dilitazem)

CARDURA (doxazosin)

CATAPRES (clonidine)

COVERA (verapamil)

COZAAR (losartan)

DILACOR (dilitazem)

DIOVAN (valsartan)

DIURIL (chlorothiazide)

HYDRODIURIL (hydrochlorothiazide [HCTZ])

HYTRIN (terazosin)

HYZAAR (losarta, HCTZ)

INDERAL (propranolol)

LASIX (furosemide)

LOPRESSOR (metoprolol)

LOTENSIN, LOTREL (benazepril)

MINIPRESS (prazosin)

MONOPRIL (fosinopril)

NORMODYNE, TRANDATE (labetalol)

NORVASC (amlodipine)

TENORMIN (atenolol)

TIAZAC (dilitazem)

TIMOLOL (blocadren)

VASOTEC (enalapril)
ZESTERIL (lisinopril)

■ Pain Management (Narcotics)

Codeine
DARVOCET-N (propoxyphene, APAP)
DARVON (propoxyphene)
DEMEROL (meperidine)
DILAUDID (hydromorphine)
DOLOPHINE (methadone)
HYDROCET (hydrocodone, APAP)
LORTAB (hydrocodone, APAP)
Morphine sulfate
MS CONTIN (morphine sulfate)
NUBAIN (nalbuphine)
OXYCONTIN (oxycodone)
PERCOCET (acetaminophen and oxycodone)
PERCODAN (oxycodone)
ROXANOL, ROXICET, ROXICODONE (morphine)
SUBLIMAZE (fentanyl)
TALWIN (pentazocine)
TYLOX (oxycodone)

■ Pain Management (Non-narcotic)

ADVIL (ibuprofen)–NSAID

AFLAXEN, ALEVE, ANAPROX (naproxen)–NSAID

APAP (acetaminophen)

Aspirin (acetylsalicylic acid)

CLINORIL (sulindac)–NSAID

DAYPRO (oxaprozin)–NSAID

FIORICET (butalbital, APAP, caffeine)–headaches

FIORINAL (butalbital, aspirin, caffeine)

FLEXARIL (cyclobenzaprine)–skeletal muscle relaxant

INDOCIN (indomethacin)–NSAID

RELAFEN (nabumetone)

TORADOL (ketorolac)

ULTRAM (tramadol)

TYLENOL (acetaminophen)

SOMA (carisoprodol)–relaxant

VOLTAREN (diclofenac)

■ Psychiatric Disorders

Antidepressants

- ANAFRANIL (clomipramine)–tricyclic
- DESYREL (trazadone)
- EFFEXOR (venlafaxine)
- ELAVIL (amitriptyline)–tricyclic

- LUVOX (fluvoxamine)
- PAMELOR (nortriptyline)–tricyclic
- REMERON (mirtazapine)
- SERZONE (nefazodone)–tricyclic
- SINEQUAN (doxepin)–tricyclic
- TOFRANIL (imipramine)
- WELBUTRIN (bupropion)

BUSPAR (buspirone)–anxiety
CLOZARIL (clozapine)–antipsychotic
ESKALITH (lithium)
HALDOL (haloperidol)
HALICON (triazolam)
Lithium carbonate (lithium)–depression, manic
MELLARIL (thioridazine)
PARNATE (tranylcpromine)–MAO inhibitor
PAXIL (paroxetine)
PROLIXIN (fluphenazine)
RISPERDAL (risperidone)
THORAZINE (chlorpromazine)–antipsychotic
TRILAFON (perphenazine)

■ Seizures

ATIVAN (lorazepam)
DEPAKENE (valproic acid)
DIASTAT

DILANTIN (phenytoin)
EPITOL (carbamazepine)
KLONOPIN (clonazepam)
LAMICTAL (lamotrigine)
MESANTOIN (mephenytoin)
MYSOLINE (primidone)
NEURONTIN (gabapentin)
SOLOFOTON (phenobarbital)
TEGRETOL (carbamazepine)
TRANXENE (clorazepate)
VALIUM (diazepam)
VERSED (short acting)

■ Stroke

PERSANTINE (dipyridamole)
TICLID (ticlopidine)

■ HIV/AIDS (Antivirals)

CRIXIVAN (indinavir)
EPIVIR (3Tc)
FAMVIR (famciclovir)
HIVID (zalcitabine)
LAMIVUDINE (3Tc)
MYCOBUTIN (rifabutin)
NORVIR (ritonavir)

RETROVIR (zidovudine)
VIRACEPT (nelfinavir)
ZERIT (D4T stavudine)
ZIDOVUDINE (AZT)
ZOVIRAX (acyclovir)

■ CNS Stimulants

ADDERALL (amphetamine)–ADD
RITALIN (methylphenidate)

■ Sleep Medicines

AMBIEN (zolpidem)
HALCION (triazolam)
RESTORIL (temazepam)

■ Antibiotics

ANCEF (cefazolin)
AMOXIL (amoxicillin)
Ampicillin
AUGMENTIN (amoxicillin clavulanate)
BACTRIM (sulfamethoxazole)
BIAXIN (clarithromycin)
CECLOR (cefaclor)
CEDAX (ceftibuten)

CEFZIL (cefprozil)
CIPRO (ciprofloxacin)
CLEOCIN (clindamycin)
Dicloxacillin
Doxycycline
DURICEF (cefadroxil)
EES (erythromycin ethylsuccinate)
Erythromycin
FLAGYL (metronidazole)
FLOXIN (ofloxacin)
Gentamycin
KEFLEX (cephalexin)
LEVAQUIN (levofloxacin)
SEPTRA (trimethoprim and sulfamethoxazole)
Tetracycline
Vancomycin
ZITHROMAX (azithromycin)

■ Cholesterol

BAYCOL (cerivastatin)
LESCOL (fluvastatin)
LIPITOR (atorvastatin)
LOPID (gemfibrozil)
MEVACOR (lovastatin)
PRAVACHOL (pravastatin)

■ Tuberculosis

INH (isoniazid)–antibiotic, tuberculosis
LEVOTHROID (levothyroxine)–thyroid
LEVOXYL (levothyroxine sodium)
SYNTHROID (levothyroxine)–thyroid
PRELONE (prednisone)–steroid
RIFADIN (rifampin, isonazid)–antibiotic,
   tuberculosis
RIFATER (pyrazinamide)–antibiotic, tuberculosis

■ Miscellaneous

ATARAX (hydroxyzine)–sedative, anxiety,
   antihistamine
BENADRYL (diphenhydramine)–allergies,
   antihistamine
Chloral hydrate–sedative
COGENTIN (benztropine)–anticholinergic,
   Parkinson's disease
FEOSOL–iron supplement
IMITREX (sumatriptan)–migraines
VERSED (midazolam)–sedative, hypnotic
XANAX (alprazolam)–sedative, hypnotic
ZYRTEC (cetirizine)–antihistamine

■ Activated Charcoal

Drug type Adsorbant

Indications/use Poisoning/overdose

Contraindications Do not give with altered LOC. Do not give with ipecac, vomiting, airway compromise, or aspiration. Contact poison center for advice.

Dosages 1 g/kg PO or NGT

Side effects Vomiting, aspiration during transport

Cautions Be prepared for vomiting or prolonged diarrhea. Prevent aspiration; position the patient.

■ Adenosine

Drug type Antiarrhythmic–tachycardia

Indications/use PSVT

Contraindications Heart blocks, bradycardia, sick sinus syndrome

Dosages 6-mg rapid IV push, lift arm, give IV flush. Repeat at 12-mg IV in 2 to 3 minutes if no response.

Side effects Brief periods of slow heart rate or even asystole. Face flush, chest pain, shortness of breath, hypotension, headache, N/V, bronchospasm

Cautions Watch cardiac monitor and recheck vital signs.

Pediatric 0.1 to 0.2 mg/kg rapid IVP

Cautions Monitor cardiac rhythm, record rhythm strip. Expect ventricular ectopy or standstill period.

■ Albuterol (Ventolin)

Drug type Bronchodilator

Indications/use Bronchospasm, asthma, COPD

Dosage 2.5 mg in 3 mL normal saline via nebulizer

Contraindications Tachycardia, how many nebulizers prior to arrival. May make symptoms worse, more congestion or coughing.

Side effects Tachycardia, anxiety, nausea and vomiting

Pediatric 0.03 mL/kg, nebulized

Cautions Be prepared to suction, clear airway. Measure SpO_2 before/after $ETco_2$.

■ Amiodarone (Cordarone)

Drug type Antiarrhythmic

Indications/use Ventricular fibrillation, ventricular tachycardia, cardiac arrest, ventricular dysrhythmias, unknown etiology wide tachycardias, atrial fibrillation

Dosage 300 mg IV; repeat at 150 mg. Drip 150 mg in 100 mL of normal saline for 10 to 20 minutes

Contraindications Bradycardias, heart blocks, cardiogenic shock

Side effects Hypotension, cardiac arrest

Cautions Check vital signs frequently, monitor ECG.

■ Aspirin (ASA)

Drug type Antiplatelet

Indications/use Heart attack, myocardial infarction, chest pain

Dosage 160 to 325 mg

Contraindications Ulcers (actively bleeding), GI bleeding, other bleeding disorders; allergy

Side effects GI bleeding

Cautions Give early if it looks like a heart attack

■ Atropine

Drug type Vagolytic, slows heart rate; orgonophosphate

Indications/use Cardiac arrest (asystole, PEA), poisoning

Dosage 0.5 to 1.0 mg; organophos: 2 to 5 mg until secretions stop

Contraindications Atrial fibrillation, atrial flutter, glaucoma

Side effects Dilated pupils, increased heart rate, dry mouth

Cautions Recheck vital signs; can be repeated.

■ Calcium Chloride

Drug type Electrolyte

Indications/use Calcium channel blocker OD, hypocalcemia, hyperkalemia

Dosage 2 to 4 mg/kg slowly over 5 minutes

Contraindications Ventricular fibrillation, digitalis toxicity, hypercalcemia

Side effects Bradycardia, asystole, hypotension, ventricular fibrillation, coronary and/or cerebral artery spasms, nausea, vomiting

Cautions May precipitate with bicarb in IV bag or tubing. Two IVs should be used.

■ Dextrose 50%

Drug type Carbohydrate (sugar)

Indications/use Unresponsive diabetes, low blood glucose

Dosage 25 g IV

Contraindications CVA, intracerebral bleeding

Side effects Tissue necrosis if IV infiltrates

Cautions May need to repeat dose or feed
patient to sustain adequate blood glucose.
Repeat blood glucose reading.

■ Diazepam (Valium)

Drug type Anticonvulsant, sedative

Indications/use Seizures, sedation

Dosage 5 to 10 mg IV slowly; may be given rectally

Contraindications Head injury, hypotension,
respiratory depression, glaucoma

Side effects Respiratory depression,
hypotension, altered mental status, vein irritation

Pediatric 0.2 mg/kg IV or IO

Cautions May need to support ventilations,
maintain airway. Check vital signs frequently.

■ Dilitiazem (Cardizem)

Drug type Antiarrhythmic

Indications/use Atrial fibrillation, atrial flutter,
PSVT

Dosage First dose, 0.25 mg/kg; no response in
15 minutes, then second dose 0.35 mg/kg slow
IV over 2 minutes

Contraindications Heart block, Hypotension, sick
sinus syndrome, Wolff-Parkinson-White syndrome

Side effects Hypotension, bradycardia, nausea and vomiting, caution with a patient taking digoxin, CHF

Cautions Frequent vital signs, monitor ECG

■ Diphenhydramine (Benadryl)

Drug type Antihistamine

Indications/use Allergic anaphyalxis, EPS reaction

Dosage 25 to 50 mg IV or IM

Contraindications Pregnancy

Side effects Sedation, blurred vision, dry mouth

Pediatric 1 to 2 mg/kg IV, IO, or IM

Cautions Takes longer if given PO, SQ

■ Dobutamine

Drug type Inotropic

Indications/use Cardiogenic shock, CHF

Dosage 2 to 20 μg/kg/min; 250 mg in 500 mL = 500 μg/mL

Contraindications Tachycardia

Side effects Tachycardia, ventricular fibrillation, HTN, myocardial infarction, nausea and vomiting

Cautions Monitor heart rate, blood pressure

DOBUTAMINE DOSAGE

Weight (kg)	Dosage 1 µg/ kg/mL	Dosage 2.5 µg/ kg/mL	Dosage 5 µg/ kg/mL	Dosage 7.5 µg/ kg/mL	Dosage 10 µg/ kg/mL	Dosage 12.5 µg/ kg/mL	Dosage 15 µg/ kg/mL	Dosage 20 µg/ kg/mL
40	4	13	24	36	48	60	70	96
45	5	14	27	41	54	68	81	108
50	6	15	30	45	60	75	90	120
55	7	17	33	50	66	83	99	132
60	7	18	36	54	72	90	108	144
65	8	20	39	59	78	98	117	156
70	8	21	42	63	84	105	126	168
75	9	23	45	68	90	113	135	180
80	10	24	48	72	96	120	144	192
85	10	26	51	77	102	128	153	204
90	11	27	54	81	108	135	162	216
100	12	30	60	90	120	150	180	240

■ Dopamine (Intropin)

Drug type Inotropic

Indications/use Cardiogenic shock, CHF

Dosage 2 to 20 µg/kg/min; mix 400 mg in
250 mL; 400 mg in 250 mL normal saline =
1,600 mg/mL

Contraindications Tachycardia

Side effects Tachycardia, causes tissue damage
if IV leaks or infiltrates

Cautions Monitor heart rate, blood pressure;
check peripheral pulses. If suspected
hypovolemia, volume should be replaced
first.

■ Epinephrine

Drug type Sympathomimetic

Indications/use Allergic reaction, anaphylaxis,
asthma, cardiac arrest

Dosage Allergic reaction: 0.3 to 0.5 mg SQ
1:1,000

Anaphylaxis: 0.3 to 0.5 mg IV 1:10,000

Cardiac arrest: 1 mg every 3 minutes

IV drip: 1 mg in 250 mL normal saline = 4 µg/mL

Contraindications Tachycardia, coronary heart
disease

DOPAMINE DOSAGE

Weight (kg)	Infusion Rate 5 µg/kg/min	Infusion Rate 10 µg/kg/min	Infusion Rate 15 µg/kg/min	Infusion Rate 20 µg/kg/min
50	9	18	28	38
55	10	20	31	41
60	11	22	34	45
65	12	24	37	49
70	13	26	39	53
75	14	28	42	56
80	15	30	45	60
85	16	32	48	64
90	17	34	51	68
95	18	36	53	71
100	19	38	56	75
105	20	39	59	79

Side effects Tachycardia, ventricular tachycardia/ventricular fibrillation, angina, HTN

Pediatric 0.01 mg/kg SQ

Cautions Caution with adults older than age 50, past medical history of CAD or HTN, monitor vital signs closely

■ Etomidate (Amidate)

Drug type Hypnotic

Indications/uses Induction of intubation, conscious sedation

Dosage 0.1 mg/kg for sedation; 0.3 mg/g for intubation

Contraindications *Must ventilate after administering to patient!*

Side effects Apnea, rigid chest involuntary muscle movements, nausea and vomiting. Short acting may have to ventilate; may need sedation.

Cautions Apply cricoid pressure to prevent regurgitation.

■ Furosemide (Lasix)

Drug type Diuretic

Indications/use CHF, pulmonary edema

Dosage 0.5 to 1.0 mg/kg IV slowly

EPINEPHRINE DOSAGE

Infusion Rate (µg/min)	Admin Set: 10 drops/mL	Admin Set: 15 drops/mL	Admin Set: 60 drops/mL
	2.5 drops/min	3.5 drops/min	15 drops/min
1	2.5		
2	5	7	30
4	10	15	60
6	15	22	90
8	20	30	120
10	25	37	150

Contraindications Dehydration, pneumonia,
hypokalemia, hypomagnesium

Side effects Hypokalemia, hypotension,
dehydration, ventricular irritability

Pediatric 1 mg/kg IV, IO slowly

Cautions Monitor blood pressure.

■ Glucagon

Drug type Increase blood glucose

Indications/use Diabetes, low blood glucose,
beta blocker, calcium channel blocker, overdoses

Dosage 0.5 to 1.0 mg IM for low blood glucose;
up to 2 mg IV drip for overdose

Contraindications Hypersensitivity

Side effects Vomiting

Pediatric 0.1 mg/kg IM or SQ up to 1 mg

Cautions Be prepared for vomiting; position
patient and make suction available.

■ Ipecac (syrup)

Drug type Induce vomiting

Indications/use Some poisonings and overdoses

Dosage 30 mL followed by one to two 8 oz
glasses of water

Contraindications Ingestion of caustic substances, petroleum products, tricyclic antidepressants, pregnancy, myocardial infarction, decreased LOC

Side effects Vomiting

Pediatric 15 mL

Cautions *Contact poison control first!*

■ Ipratropium (Atrovent)

Drug type Anticholinergic, prevents bronchospasms

Indications/use Poisoning, overdose

Dosage 0.5 mg in 2.5 mL normal saline, usually with albuterol

Contraindications Inhalation aerosol is contraindicated in patients with a history of hypersensitivity to soy lecithin or related food products, such as soybean and peanut. Tachycardia.

Side effects Tachycardia, tremors, nervousness, nausea, and vomiting

■ Ketorolac (Toradol)

Drug type NSAID pain relief

Indications/use Pain management

Dosage 15 to 30 mg; 30-60 mg IM

Contraindications Allergy to aspirin, NSAIDS; caution with liver and renal diseases, COPD, asthma, ulcers, bleeding disorders, coumadin use, elderly

Side effects Nausea, GI bleeding, edema

■ Lidocaine

Drug type Antiarrhythmic

Indications/use Cardiac arrest, prepare for RSI

Dosage 1 to 1.5 mg/kg, repeat in 8 to 10 minutes; max 3 mg/kg

100 mg of lidocaine in 100 mL normal saline + 2 mg/mL

LIDOCAINE DOSAGE

Infusion Rate (mg/min)	Admin Set: 60 drops/mL
1	30 drops/min
2	60
3	90
4	120

Contraindications Heart blocks, hypotension

Side effects Sedation, seizures, slurred speech, altered mental status

Cautions Use in elderly, liver disease, CHF or shock. Check vital signs; monitor GCS and ECG

■ Lorazepam (Ativan)

Drug type Anticonvulsant, sedative

Indications/use Seizures

Dosage 2 to 4 mg slow IV or IM

Contraindications Acute narrow-angle glaucoma

Side effects Apnea, N/V, altered LOC, restless, hypotension

Dosage For IV or IO use, dilute 1:1 normal saline. An overdose may be reversed with Flumazenil.

Cautions *Be prepared to ventilate.* May need to support ventilations, maintain airway. Check vital signs frequently.

■ Magnesium Sulfate

Drug type Antiarrhythmic, electrolyte

Indications/use Seizures, eclampsia, ventricular fibrillation/ventricular tachycardia, torsade de pointes, ventricular ectopy

Dosage 1 to 4 g IV over 1 minute for eclampsia; 1 to 2 g IV over 1 to 2 minutes for torsade de pointes

Contraindications Heart blocks, renal disease

Side effects Respiratory depression, decreased reflexes, hypotension, cardiac arrest

Cautions Monitor ECG, recheck vital signs frequently

■ **Metoprolol (Lopressor)**

Drug type Anti-anginal, HTN, antiarrhythmic

Indications/use ST elevation myocardial infarction, ACS chest pain

Dosage 5 mg every 5 minutes × 3, *if* heart rate is > 60 beats/min

Contraindications Heart blocks, bradycardia, sick sinus syndrome, severe CHF, cardiogenic shock

Side effects Dizziness, decreased heart rate, hypotension, nausea and vomiting, difficulty breathing

Cautions Monitor ECG, recheck vital signs frequently, assist with 12-lead ECG.

■ **Midazolam (Versed)**

Drug type Anticonvulsant, sedative

Indications/use Seizures, sedation

Dosage 0.05 mg/kg IV or IM; may repeat

Contraindications Acute narrow-angle glaucoma, hypotension, shock

Side effects Apnea, N/V, altered LOC, hypotension

Cautions Be prepared to ventilate! May need to support ventilations, maintain airway. Check vital signs frequently.

■ Morphine Sulfate

Drug type Analgesic, opioid

Indications/use Pain management, pulmonary edema

Dosage 0.05 mg/kg IV or IM; may repeat. For IV or IO use, dilute 1:1 normal saline. Overdose may be reversed with Narcan.

Contraindications Head injury, exacerbated COPD, respiratory depression, hypotension, altered LOC, caution with undiagnosed abdominal pain

Side effects Apnea, N/V, altered LOC, restlessness, hypotension

Cautions Be prepared to ventilate! May need to support ventilations, maintain airway. Check vital signs frequently.

■ Naloxone (Narcan)

Drug type Narcotic antagonist

Indications/use Opiate overdose, coma

Dosage 1 to 2 mg slow IV, IM, ETT

Contraindications Fast IVP may precipitate ventricular fibrillation

Side effects Withdrawal symptoms, agitation, violent behavior (anticipate rapid onset)

■ Nitroglycerin

Drug type Vasodilator

Indications/use Angina, myocardial infarction, pulmonary edema

Dosage 0.4 mg SL; repeat every 3 to 5 minutes *if* blood pressure is > 90.

Contraindications Hypotension, hypovolemia, intracranial bleeding. RV/posterior infarct use with caution

Side effects Headache, bitter taste, hypotension, syncope tachycardia, flush

Cautions Monitor blood pressure; recheck vital signs frequently.

■ Procainamide (Pronestyl)

Drug type Antiarrhythmic

Indications/use Supraventricular tachycardia/
Wolff-Parkinson-White syndrome, refractory
ventricular fibrillation or ventricular tachycardia

Dosage 20 to 30 mg/min IV until the rhythm is
converted, hypotension, QT widens/prolongs, or
17 mg/kg has been given

Contraindications Heart block, torsade de
pointes, digitalis toxicity

Side effects QT widening, AV block, cardiac
arrest, hypotension, N/V

Cautions Monitor ECG; recheck vital signs
frequently.

■ Sodium Bicarbonate

Drug type Alkalinizer

Indications/use Cardiac arrest, metabolic
acidosis, tricyclic overdose

Dosage 1 mEq/kg; repeat 0.5 mEq

Contraindications *Must ventilate after
administering to patient!*

Side effects Alkalosis, decreased potassium

Cautions *Must ventilate after administering to
patient!*

■ Succinylcholine (Anectine)

Drug type Paralytic

Indications/uses Paralysis to facilitate
intubation

Dosage 1 to 2 mg/kg IV; wait 90 seconds for effect

Contraindications Acute glaucoma, penetrating
eye injuries, burns older than 8 hours, massive
crush injury/syndrome, conditions with high
potassium

Side effects Apnea, malignant hyperthermia
(Dannitrol–notify hospital early), arrhythmias,
HTN, tachycardia

Cautions Assess mid-face stability prior to use;
ensure ability to ventilate prior to use; apply
cricoid pressure to prevent regurgitation.

■ Vecuronium (Norcuron)

Drug type Paralytic

Indications/uses Paralysis to facilitate
intubation

Dosage 0.01 mg/kg IV defaciculating dose;
0.1 mg IVP maintenance of paralysis. Wait for
effect 90 seconds, effect lasts from 45 to 60
minutes.

Contraindications Newborns, myasthenia gravis

Side effects Apnea, profound weakness

Medication Formulary

Cautions Assess mid-face stability prior to use. Ensure ability to ventilate prior to use. Ensure endotracheal tube placement verification prior to administration. Continue to apply cricoid pressure to prevent regurgitation.

■ Pediatric Broselow Scale

PEDIATRIC BROSELOW SCALE

Weight (kg)	Equipment Needed
3 to 5	O_2 mask: Pediatric NRB Oral airway: 50 mm Nasal airway: 14F Suction catheter: 8F Bag-mask device: Infant/Child BP cuff: Neonatal, #5/Infant IV access: 22 to 24 gauge IO access: 18 to 15 gauge ET tube size: 3.0 uncuffed Laryngoscope: 1 straight
6 to 9	O_2 mask: Pediatric NRB Oral airway: 50 mm Nasal airway: 14F Suction catheter: 8F Bag-mask device: Infant/Child BP cuff: Infant/Child IV access: 22 to 24 gauge IO access: 18 to 15 gauge ET tube size: 3.5 uncuffed Laryngoscope: 1 straight

PEDIATRIC BROSELOW SCALE (*cont.*)

Weight (kg)	Equipment Needed
10 to 11	O$_2$ mask: Pediatric NRB Oral airway: 60 mm Nasal airway: 18F Suction catheter: 10F Bag-mask device: Child BP cuff: Child IV access: 20 to 24 gauge IO access: 15 gauge ET tube size: 4.0 uncuffed Laryngoscope: 1 straight
12 to 14	O$_2$ mask: Pediatric NRB Oral airway: 60 mm Nasal airway: 20F Suction catheter: 10F Bag-mask device: Child BP cuff: Child IV access: 18 to 22 gauge IO Access 15 gauge ET tube size: 4.5 uncuffed Laryngoscope: 2 straight
15 to 18	O$_2$ mask: Pediatric NRB Oral airway: 60 mm Nasal airway: 20F Suction catheter: 10F

PEDIATRIC BROSELOW SCALE *(cont.)*

Weight (kg)	Equipment Needed
15 to 18	Bag-mask device: Child BP cuff: Child IV access: 18 to 22 gauge IO access: 15 gauge ET tube size: 5.0 uncuffed Laryngoscope: 2 straight
19 to 23	O$_2$ mask: Pediatric NRB Oral airway: 70 mm Nasal airway: 24F Suction catheter: 10F Bag-mask device: Child BP cuff: Child IV access: 18 to 20 gauge IO access: 15 gauge ET tube size: 5.5 uncuffed Laryngoscope: 2 straight/curved
24 to 29	O$_2$ mask: Pediatric NRB Oral airway: 80 mm Nasal airway: 26F Suction catheter: 10F Bag-mask device: Child BP cuff: Child

Quick Reference

PEDIATRIC BROSELOW SCALE (cont.)

Weight (kg)	Equipment Needed
24 to 29	IV access: 18 to 20 gauge
	IO access: 15 gauge
	ET tube size: 6.0 cuffed
	Laryngoscope: 2 straight/curved
30 to 36	O_2 mask: Pediatric/Adult NRB
	Oral airway: 80 mm
	Nasal airway: 30F
	Suction catheter: 10F to 12F
	Bag-mask device: Adult
	BP cuff: Small Adult
	IV access: 16 to 20 gauge
	IO access: 15 gauge
	ET tube size: 6.5 cuffed
	Laryngoscope: 3 straight/curved

■ Glasgow Coma Scale
GLASGOW COMA SCALE (ADULT/PEDIATRIC)

Infant	Child/Adult
Eye opening:	
4–Spontaneously	4–Spontaneously
3–To speech	3–To speech
2–To pain	2–To pain
1–No response	1–No response
Best verbal response:	
5–Coos, babbles	5–Oriented
4–Irritable, cries	4–Confused
3–Cries to pain words	3–Inappropriate
2–Moans, grunts	2–Incomprehensible
1–No response	1–No response
Best motor response:	
6–Spontaneous	6–Obeys command
5–Localizes pain	5–Localizes pain
4–Withdraw pain	4–Withdraw pain
3–Flexion	3–Flexion
2–Extension	2–Extension
1–No response	1–No response
Total:	_____

(GCS < 8 = Intubate)

■ Common Abbreviations

Abd	abdomen
A&O	alert and oriented
ASA	aspirin
ASHD	arteriosclerotic heart disease
bid	twice a day
BM	bowel movement
BSA	body surface area
BVM	bag-valve-mask
$\bar{c}$	with
CA	cancer
CABG	coronary artery bypass graft
CAD	coronary artery disease
CAP	capsule
CBC	complete blood count
CC	chief complaint
cc	cubic centimeter
CHF	congestive heart failure
CID	cervical immobilization device
cm	centimeter
CNS	central nervous system
CO	carbon monoxide
CO_2	carbon dioxide
COPD	chronic obstructive pulmonary disease
CSF	cerebrospinal fluid

CVA	cerebrovascular accident (stroke)
d/c	discontinue
DKA	diabetic ketoacidosis
DNR	do not resuscitate
DOB	date of birth
Dx	diagnosis
ET	endotracheal
ETA	estimated time of arrival
ETOH	Alcohol
GCS	Glascow Coma Scale
GI	gastrointestinal
GSW	gunshot wound
gt	drop
gtt	drops
GU	genitourinary
HIV	human immunodeficiency virus (AIDS)
HR	heart rate
hr	hour
HTN	hypertension (high blood pressure)
Hx	history
IM	intramuscular
inj	injection; injury
IO	intraosseous
IV	intravenous
JVD	jugular vein distention

K	potassium
kg	kilogram
Ⓛ	left
L	liter
LBB	long backboard
LLQ	left lower quadrant
LMP	last menstrual period
LOC	level of consciousness or loss of consciousness
lpm	liters per minute
LUQ	left upper quadrant
m	meter
m	minimum
MCI	multiple casualty incident
mg	milligram
mcg, μg	microgram
MI	myocardial infarction (heart attack)
min	minute or minimum
mL	milliliter
mm	millimeter
MOI	mechanism of injury
Na	sodium
NC	nasal cannula
neg	negative
NOI	nature of illness
NTG	nitroglycerin

N&V	nausea and vomiting
O_2	oxygen
OB	obstetrics
OBS	organic brain syndrome
OD	overdose or right eye
OS	left eye
OTC	over-the-counter
OU	both eyes
p̄	after
PAT	paroxysmal atrial tachycardia
PCN	penicillin
PE	physical exam or pulmonary embolism
PID	pelvic inflammatory disease
PO	by mouth
prn	as needed
Pt	patient
PVC	premature ventricular contraction
Px	physical examination
q	every
qAM	every morning
qd	every day
qh	every hour
q2h	every 2 hours
q3h	every 3 hours
q4h	every 4 hours

q6h	every 6 hours
q12h	every 12 hours
qid	four times daily
qod	every other day
qPM	every night
®	right
RBC	red blood count or cell
RLQ	right lower quadrant
R/O	rule out
RUQ	right upper quadrant
Rx	medication or prescription
SC	subcutaneous
s̄	without
SL	sublingual
SOB	short of breath
SQ	subcutaneous
TAB	tablet
temp	temperature
TIA	transient ischemic attack
tid	three times daily
top	topical
Tx	treatment
UTI	urinary tract infection
VF	ventricular fibrillation
VS	vital signs
VT	ventricular tachycardia
WBC	white blood count or cell

w/	with
w/o	without
wk	week
wt	weight
yr	year

Adult Protective Services	_____
Air Medical Service	_____
AIDS Information	_____
Alzheimer's Information	_____
American Red Cross	_____
Animal Control	_____
Battered Women's Hotline	1-800-424-9300
CHEMTREC	_____
Children's Services	_____
CISM Team	_____
Communications/Dispatch	_____
Domestic Violence Center	_____
Hazardous Materials Team	_____
Health Department	_____
Homeless Shelter	_____
Infection Control Department	_____
Medical Examiner/Coroner	1-800-625-3780
Medic Alert	_____
Poison/Drug Information Center	_____
Psychiatric Emergency Services	_____
Rape/Sexual Abuse Crisis Center	_____
SIDS Hotline	_____
Suicide Prevention Hotline	_____
Towing Service/Heavy Wrecker	_____
Translators (Note Language)	_____
Toxicologist	_____

HOSPITAL PHONE NUMBERS AND RADIO CHANNELS

Hospital Name	Medical Control Phone Number	Emergency Room Phone Number	Med Radio Channel

Note—If the hospital has a dedicated phone number for contacting medical control, note this in the appropriate space. Otherwise, leave blank and use the regular emergency room phone number for communications. If the hospital has medical radio capability, note which radio channel to use.

Quick Reference